MEDICINE BALL
WORKOUTS

MEDICINE BALL
WORKOUTS

Strengthen Major and Supporting
Muscle Groups for Increased Power,
Coordination and Core Stability

BRETT STEWART

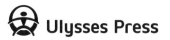 Ulysses Press

Published in the United States by
Ulysses Press
P.O. Box 3440
Berkeley, CA 94703
www.ulyssespress.com

ISBN13: 978-1-61243-130-7
Library of Congress Control Number 2012951890

Printed in Canada by Marquis Book Printing

10 9 8 7 6 5 4 3 2 1

Acquisitions Editor: Keith Riegert
Managing Editor: Claire Chun
Editor: Lily Chou
Proofreader: Elyce Berrigan-Dunlop
Cover design: whatldesign @ whatweb.com
Production: Jake Flaherty
Cover photographs: front © MichaelSvoboda/istockphoto.com; back © Scott Whitney
Models: Lewis Elliot, Tricia Schafer, Brett Stewart, Kristen Stewart and Jason Warner

Distributed by Publishers Group West

Please Note: This book has been written and published strictly for informational purposes, and in no way should be used as a substitute for consultation with health care professionals. You should not consider educational material herein to be the practice of medicine or to replace consultation with a physician or other medical practitioner. The author and publisher are providing you with information in this work so that you can have the knowledge and can choose, at your own risk, to act on that knowledge. The author and publisher also urge all readers to be aware of their health status and to consult health care professionals before beginning any health program.

To my kids, Vivi & Ian—you are stronger, smarter and more talented than you may ever imagine. When you believe in yourself, anything is possible.
—Dad

CONTENTS

PART 1: OVERVIEW

Introduction

When it comes to fitness, nutrition or competition I abide by one rule: Only do it if it makes you happy. Of course, happiness is relative, and a series of medicine ball toss-and-sprints will surely make me happier than the lady from Human Resources dropping off a stack of employee reviews that need to be done before the end of the week, right?

Interestingly enough, the above example is exactly the type of situation that got me started in medicine ball workouts. I was the director of engineering for a technology start-up and spent five days (or more) a week plopped behind a desk filling out paperwork, dealing with software development issues or attending meetings about meetings where we'd discuss why we didn't accomplish what we talked about last meeting. Usually, the answer was to put together another meeting with the stakeholders. Buzz words abounded, but extremely little progress was made. Someone would "ping" someone about "synergies" and we'd all brainstorm about who the hell knows what for our "version 2.0" product and, before we knew it, the whole engineering team was a bunch of jaded zombies showing up for a paycheck and desperately trying to get through each mind-

numbingly boring day with as little interaction with everyone else as possible. Does this sound like your workplace?

Well, Jason Warner (my co-author on *Ultimate Jump Rope Workouts* and *7 Weeks to 10 Pounds of Muscle*) and I decided enough was enough and if we couldn't change the working atmosphere inside the office, we were going to take full advantage of every second before the morning commute, at lunchtime and immediately after work. A huge advantage of working with your best friend and workout partner is the built-in motivation from being around someone who is pushing to reach their goals, no matter how different those goals may be from your own. Jason is all about strength; he's 4 inches taller and 60 pounds heavier than me and loves lifting weights, packing on muscle, playing rugby and all that burly-man stuff. As a

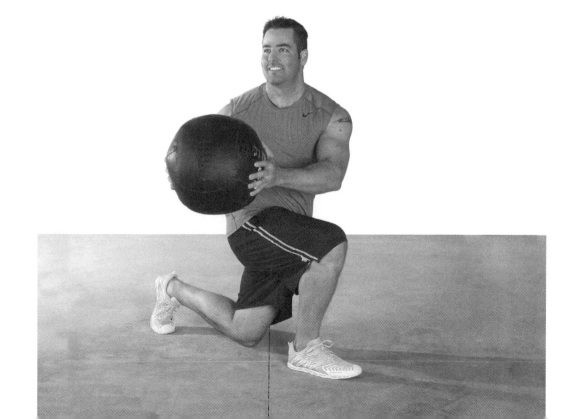

runner and triathlete, my main focus is on being light, fast and lean. What, you may ask, did we have in common? Medicine ball workouts.

Medicine balls combined the best of both worlds for our workouts—they're light enough that a small guy like me could sprint carrying one over my head and heavy enough that a big guy like Jason could single-leg shot-put it 20 yards. With just an 8-pound medicine ball we'd picked up at a local sporting goods store for less than $40, we came up with dozens of different games, exercises and routines that nearly anyone can perform. Before work we'd meet at the park by my house for our morning toss-and-sprint drills; at lunchtime we'd head over to the soccer fields near our office in Scottsdale, Arizona, and challenge each other at cross-ball or a multitude of other games before working on our long-distance tosses.

After a few weeks of coming back to the office with a renewed passion and vigor to tackle the rest of the day, more and more co-workers started to join us—and we needed to purchase a few more medicine balls! The influx of more workout partners led to the creation of new routines to get us all involved. It didn't hurt that a few of them are absolute geniuses too! After we punched out of the office we'd hit the field again for some core work before our 30-minute commute back home. During the drive, we'd usually talk about other exercises, drills or games we could try the following day. What can we say, we're fitness geeks.

All of this relates directly back to my singular rule of workout happiness. I greatly enjoyed the workouts and the camaraderie, and surely loved the results of being fit, fast and strong—all thanks to a medicine ball!

About the Book

It should come as no surprise that this book is about using a medicine ball to develop strength, total-body fitness and a shredded physique. If you're shocked by this revelation, please flip back to the cover and check the title: *Medicine Ball Workouts*.

The goal of this book is to show dozens of different exercises, tosses, games and drills you can perform by yourself or with workout partners that will take your fitness, strength, speed, endurance and flexibility to new levels—all while having fun. Most of the routines, drills, games and movements are simple and repeatable enough for you to get a quick workout in less than 20 minutes almost anywhere, provided you have some space and a medicine ball!

PART I is designed to answer all your questions about why you'd choose this type of workout, what size and weight ball to buy and other frequently asked questions. We'll also cover how to prepare for your workout, the importance of warming up and stretching, some precautions to take before you start any strenuous workout of this type and setting your fitness goals.

PART II features the Basic and Advanced programs. It also offers some tips on your next steps after completing the programs.

PART III features a bevy of exercises, games, tosses and drills, which you can use to make up your own routine. With the mindset of getting fit and having fun while doing it, this section should be the go-to resource for your fitness regimen for years to come.

THE APPENDIX contains warm-ups and stretches to complement your workout.

What Is a Medicine Ball?

A medicine ball is also known as an exercise ball, a med ball or a fitness ball, not to be confused with an inflatable exercise ball, a physio ball, a stability ball or a buffoon ball. (OK, I made up that last one—just trying to have a little fun with all these redundant names.)

Quite simply, a medicine ball is a weighted sphere roughly between 12 and 20 inches in diameter that's designed to provide additional muscle activation during exercise movements. Contemporary medicine balls are normally covered in rubber or leather, while the earliest examples date back to around 1000 B.C., when they were animal hides filled with sand and sewn together and used by gladiators.

The term "medicine" in reference to the weighted exercise ball can be dated back to a Renaissance doctor who prescribed their use for "medicinal gymnastics." The terms "medicine" and "health" were indeed more synonymous than they are today, and apparently the name stuck.

Now, to complicate things a bit, there are many variations of medicine balls that are used for a multitude of training. We'll cover the following in this book:

Rubber-coated, basketball-sized balls are 9 inches in diameter and weigh from 4 to 25 pounds. They can be used for tosses and exercise movements and are not intended to be thrown and caught. Some variations are designated "slam balls" and are designed to absorb the impact when hitting the floor or wall, not bounce back toward you.

Rubber-coated, volleyball-sized balls are slightly heavier: 10 to 12 inches in diameter and weigh from 30 to 60 pounds. They can also be used for tosses and exercise movements and are not intended to be thrown and caught.

Leather- or durable-fabric-covered balls are beach ball–sized, 14 to 20 inches in diameter and weigh 10 to 30 pounds. These are larger and softer than a rubber-coated ball and designed for tossing to a partner or throwing up and catching to minimize risk of injury. These are also referred to as "classic" or "boxing medicine balls" and have very distinguishing laces holding the ball together.

Medicine balls with one or more handles can be used for myriad medicine ball exercises and tosses. In addition, due to their shape, they can be used to perform kettlebell-like movements.

Medicine balls with a mooring point for a rope can be used for swings, momentum tosses and wall- or floor-slam exercises.

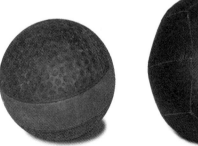
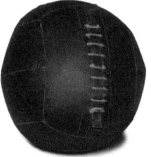
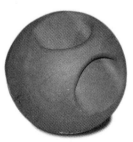

Rubber-coated   *Leather*   *With handles*

Why Use a Medicine Ball?

There's a reason why nearly all sports are based around a ball. The spherical shape allows for multiple hand placement for lifting, tossing and catching in play, and also makes the perfect object for strength training or optimal sports performance. Speaking of sports, the irony is not lost on me that a bowling ball, used by some of the least-fit professional athletes on the planet, is more akin to a medicine ball than the footballs used by modern gladiators of the gridiron. It just doesn't seem to add up, right? Well, enough about that.

Medicine balls can be found throughout history for fitness conditioning and injury rehabilitation. Hippocrates, the "father of medicine," had his patients throw weighted spheres back and forth for injury prevention, strengthening, conditioning and rehabilitation. The U.S. Military Academy at West Point has used them for more than 200 years, and they were considered to be one of the most important tools to physically prepare soldiers for battle until the late 1960s and '70s ushered in a new affinity for cardio that quickly found its way into military training programs. Luckily, what's old is new again, and the armed forces have found that bodyweight exercises augmented by medicine ball lifts, twists and tosses are incrementally more beneficial than running and basic calisthenics are alone.

Adding weights to the already efficient full-body workout provided by bodyweight exercises enhances the effectiveness of calisthenics as a strength-training regimen—to which medicine balls are the perfect accompaniment! Portable, inexpensive, effective and widely adaptable to most exercises, games and tosses, medicine balls are quite possibly the best tool for developing total-body strength, flexibility and all-around fitness.

Aside from being able to be tossed, rolled and used in games, medicine balls are more effective than dumbbells or barbells in any exercise where the weight has the potential of coming in contact with your body, floor or, well, anything else! Rubberized or leather balls do far less damage when accidentally dropped on a foot, bumped into your head and especially when landing on wood or tile flooring. As you'll see throughout the exercises in this book, if you want to use a medicine ball to curl, press, toss, catch or to perform push-ups on or even lift with your feet during pull-ups, then balance, skill and proprioception are required. Some of these moves could possibly be done with a dumbbell, and one or two may allow an awkward barbell rep or two, but all the exercises can be performed fluidly and safely with one friendly and inexpensive medicine ball.

How to Use a Medicine Ball

If you've ever picked up a basketball or volleyball, all but the largest and heaviest of medicine balls shouldn't be too much of a surprise when you first grab one. Normally, rubber-coated balls are textured to provide plenty of grip and many of the high-tech newer models feature dimples and patterns to enhance the tactile experience. Larger and heavier leather ones may take a little getting used to, but those should be handled once you've developed a little more experience, dexterity and strength.

Using a medicine ball with common calisthenics can make them even more effective as a strength-training routine. Medicine ball sit-ups activate and strengthen more core muscles, throw in a twist to invite your obliques to the party and boom—you've upgraded one familiar move into a core-blasting technique. Push-ups, pull-ups, squats, burpees and many more everyday bodyweight exercises can get kicked up a notch or two by adding a medicine ball. This helps you develop a stronger, fitter body in even less time than without!

Tossing a medicine ball is primarily done to develop core strength, flexibility, sport-specific ability, total-body power and coordination. Examples of tosses include exploding from a squatting stance and throwing the ball over your head as far as you can behind you, kneeling and pushing the ball out from your chest for maximum distance, shot-put, etc.

One of the early uses of medicine balls will not be covered in this book, and that's tossing or dropping a medicine ball on a training partner's abdomen to simulate a punch and strengthen abdominal muscles by concussive force. Common among boxers and MMA fighters, this type of medicine ball usage is outside the scope of this book and was consciously omitted. Aside from controlled tosses and a few games, we're focusing on exercises where the intention is to not let the ball impact either you or your training partner.

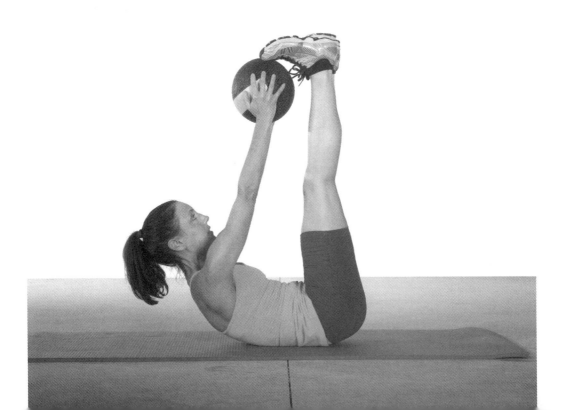

Frequently Asked Questions

Q. *What type/size/weight should I use?*

A. Well, it depends on how big your hands are, how strong you are and what your fitness goals are. This multi-part question requires at least a few answers, and is a common one I receive all the time. Experienced athletes looking to build strength while developing sports-specific proficiency should opt for the heaviest balls they can handle, while individuals looking to develop their flexibility and tone their physique are best served by easier-to-handle, lighter balls. For the most part, the exercises found in this book can be performed with any of the medicine balls listed in the table on page 14. The easiest to obtain and usually the least expensive are the first two on that list (9-, 10- or 11-inch models), and they're normally available in weights ranging from 4 to 25 pounds. You can find them at most large sporting goods stores.

If your budget allows, it surely doesn't hurt to have a few different weights, as you may be able to perform some exercises like the wood chop (page 57) with a heavier ball than you can use to knock out sets of mason twists (page 73). Also, some complicated tosses like the single-leg shot-put (page 95) require a lighter weight to get the hang of it before moving on to a heavier medicine ball.

Q. *If I were to buy just one medicine ball to use for all the exercises in this book, which would you recommend?*

A. If the answer to the last question didn't help you sort it out, then I'll use the most worn-out medicine balls in my own gym to help you decide. From experience, I've found that an 8-pound ball is great for guys to perform most exercises, tosses and games, and the 6-pounder is the medicine ball of choice for most women. Handles are surely helpful and provide the ability to perform kettlebell-like exercises as well as fling them wicked far for some tosses.

Q. *What should I wear?*

A. If you're performing these exercises in the confines of your own home, then wear as little or as much as you'd like. Comfortable athletic clothing that will let you squat, jump and twist in all directions is recommended. Since you'll be on the floor or ground for some moves, make sure your clothing is appropriate for the surface you'll be lying on. Lastly, shoes are really important as many moves will require solid footing and shoes may also provide a teeny bit of protection if you happen to misjudge a toss and drop a ball on your toes.

Q. *How long is this workout?*

From warm-up to finish, I like to make my workouts less than 45 minutes for strength training and conditioning. Multiple reports have shown that after about that point, free testosterone in your system begins to decrease and your gains decrease rapidly while the risk of overtraining increases. Keep it simple: Warm up, work out, cool down, go on with your life.

Q. *Can I do this workout every day?*

A. You can, but you shouldn't. Hitting the same muscles repeatedly within a 24-hour period has the potential of doing a lot more harm than good. This is called overtraining. While the term almost has a braggadocio to it ("I'm so fit I can overtrain"), the effects are nothing to brag about. Chronically sore muscles that have no chance to recover in between workouts not only don't grow bigger, they're more susceptible to tears and long-term deep-tissue damage. The workouts in this book were created to be performed three days a week, with at least one day of rest between workouts, so you can recover mentally and physically. The last thing I want is for you to feel like these workouts are a boring drain of your time—then you'll never stick it out and hit your goals!

Q. *How can I find time for a workout? I walk to work, uphill both ways, in the snow, without boots...*

A. Yes, we all have real life to keep us busy and it can be difficult to sneak a workout in on a regular basis. Actually, YOU are the one making it difficult. Yeah, I'm pointing my finger squarely at you, and defy you to prove me wrong. Without any question, you have 15–20 minutes to spare three times a week to improve your physique and feel better about yourself and you know it's true. Wake up a few minutes earlier, go to bed a few minutes later, cut down on your TV-watching or web-surfing and you'll be surprised how easy it is to make sure you don't miss a quick workout. If you need some help remembering, set a calendar reminder or use a mobile app like the one I made as a companion to this book (shameless plug). The bottom line is: You can find the time quite easily if you want to, and you want to, right?

Tip: Work out for half of your lunch break three days a week. If you get an hour, use 30 minutes to warm up, work out, cool down and clean up and you'll still have plenty of time to eat the (healthy) lunch that you packed. It only takes a little planning to make this work, so make it happen!

Q. *What's this "rest" thing you keep talking about? Have you seen my schedule?*

A. If you don't rest, you won't recover. If you don't recover, you lose most of the benefit from your workout. I use the term "most" because you still burned some extra calories during the exercise and raised your heart rate to obtain some cardiovascular conditioning benefit...but if you don't rest well, you'll miss out on the benefits of building lean muscle.

Q. *What are the benefits of building lean muscle?*

A. Wow, what a perfect segue from the previous question! Aside from the obvious aesthetic benefits of having a muscular physique, building lean muscle is one of those "gifts that keep giving": the more lean muscle you have, the more calories your body will naturally burn throughout the day to keep your awesome physique, well, awesome. Lean muscle not only acts like a furnace for burning calories and fat, but it also makes the muscles that you have even more adept at growing by stimulating insulin and testosterone development. (Yes, this is a ridiculously simple overview of your body's biomechanics and energy systems, but this is just an FAQ, not a PhD dissertation.) Lean muscle is a good thing, cool?

Q. *My buddy/the guy at the gym/my mother's co-worker Dawn said I should do Workout X and I'll be the fittest person on the planet! Why don't you just show me a shortcut to fitness like Workout X, huh? Are you trying to hide something?!*

A. Step 1: Chill. Out.

Step 2. Repeat Step 1.

I'll let you in on a little secret: Every workout is the best ever, provided you stick to it and get the results you want. I've developed and tested hundreds of my own different programs. Along the way I've tried out many of the big-name programs that you see online and even on late-night TV with varying levels of success. Some I like quite a bit to this day and others I'm glad I tried out just once. There are a million different ways to work out—the best way to learn what works for you is to give new exercise routines a shot. Not only will you add to your repertoire of exercises, you'll be hitting some muscles in new and exciting ways and getting fitter along the way. I like to view getting—and staying—fit as a journey: Take it all in and try some new stuff. You never know what you'll learn along the way!

Q. *I have an injury. Can I still work out?*

A. See your doctor. Boring answer, but the truth. The workouts are rigorous and the addition of a medicine ball could make some very common injuries worse if you're not careful. Above all else, be safe and see your doctor first before performing any demanding physical activity.

Q. *I already work out at the gym. Would I get anything out of this?*

A. Absolutely! The exercises and workouts here would make anyone a fitter person, not to mention a better athlete. Who can't use a stronger core, more balanced and stable musculature and better body awareness?

Q. *I want to tone up. Won't weights make me bulky?*

A. No. Absolutely not. This is a common fear for women and endurance athletes who want to stay as light as possible while developing muscle tone. Ask anyone working out in the gym just how hard it is to get the "bulky" look. Most people lifting weights crave bigger muscles, yet so few achieve it. Why? Diet. Muscle size is more a function of what and how you eat and not how you work out. Weights are the key to a healthy lifestyle, but how big you get depends on how much of the various macronutrients you eat. No, lifting weights without following a specific muscle-building nutrition plan won't make you bulky at all.

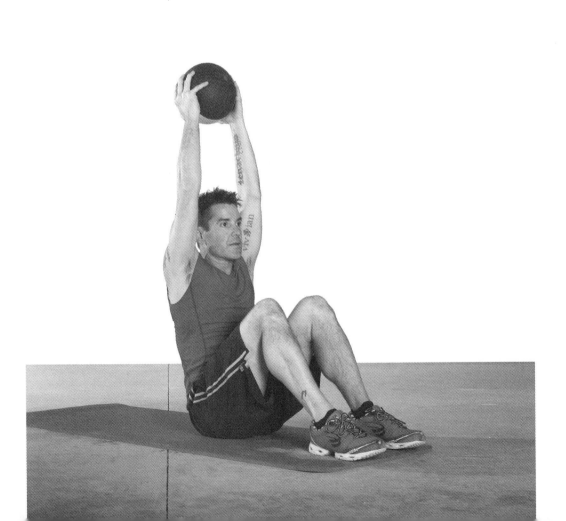

Before You Begin

If I haven't beaten you over the head with the "see your doctor first before starting any workout program" phrasing, let's just give you five practical examples of why seeing a doctor first is the most important step toward getting in shape:

1. You may be in better shape than you realize—it happens every day. How many times do you hear a co-worker say, "I got a clean bill of health. My doc says I have the heart of a teenager!"

2. You may find out you have to switch your goals and fix a potential problem. Let's face it, humans were given brains in order to solve things—we love to fix stuff. Your doctor may give you some professional insight into some fixes that your body may need, whether proactively to prevent something or reactively to take care of now. Do you know your cholesterol levels? Do you even know what they should be? How about your blood pressure, lung and heart function? All these are very easy things for a trained medical professional to test for—this is why they're professionals!

3. Use your doctor's visit as a chance to play show and tell. No, wait, that's a bad idea. How about using your visit as a chance for some Q&A? Engage your doc and ask some of the questions from #2 above. Ask what your weight should be, things you should be aware of based on your medical history and that of your family. She's the one with the clipboard in her hand. Many times there are answers in there that you need to ask for. Be vocal—you're the one paying for the visit! Your health and well-being are your responsibility,

and sometimes you won't get that extra bit of important information unless you ask.

4. There could be something serious that you can't ignore. It's the elephant in the room but it needs to be said. You need to know if there's anything wrong BEFORE you push yourself. Humans are messy and complicated, just like the wiring of a 1962 Jaguar E-Type. Both require being brought to a professional to decipher, diagnose and repair.

5. It may prevent you from spinning your wheels while trying to reach your goals. Can't gain muscle or lose weight no matter how hard you try? The problem may be no bigger than the tip of your pinkie finger. Your pituitary gland's function may be out of whack. Maybe your thyroid is operating at hyper- or hypothyroid levels? Are you anemic? What about any other vitamin deficiencies? The answer is most likely hidden inside of you and you just don't know until you get checked out. Go to a professional and decode your own internal DaVinci Code.

One last time for the lawyers: Prior to beginning this or any physical fitness regimen, it's recommended that you visit a licensed physician and receive a clean bill of health before you proceed.

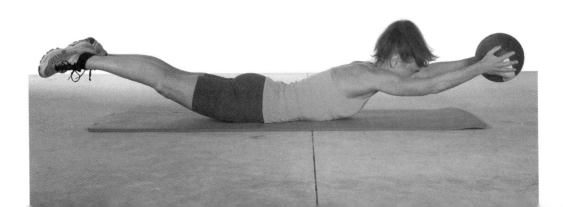

Preparing for the Workouts

Before we get on (or lift) the ball, let's cover some anatomical terms, tips and body positions that will be used in the exercise descriptions. No one's going to test you on correct use of any of the terms, but it's really helpful to have a general idea. This is barely more in-depth than the "foot bone's connected to the ankle bone..." song—it's just a few points of reference.

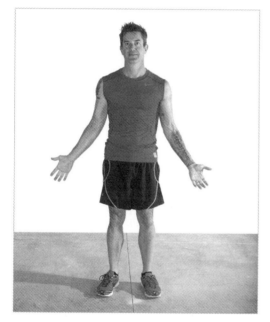

Anatomical Position: This is essentially the "default position" for your body as nearly all joints are in neutral position with the exception of your elbows (which are rotated forward to bring your palms onto the frontal plane)—feet face forward and are about shoulder-width apart, spine is erect, arms are extended at the sides of your trunk with palms facing forward. The three different anatomical planes of movement are median, frontal and horizontal, and all are described by starting with the anatomical position. Median plane splits your body laterally into right and left halves with a line vertical to your belly button (the medial line). Frontal plane splits your body into a front (anterior) and back (posterior) from the side, bisecting your torso vertically in a line that runs through your ears, shoulders, hips and ankles. Horizontal plane splits your body into upper (superior) and lower (inferior) halves at your belly button. Most motions in life are a combination of these planes.

Athletic Position: Similar to anatomical position, this is often described as "ready position" for many sports or training. I'll refer to this in nearly every exercise where you're on your feet. In a standing position, your feet face forward and are approximately shoulder-width apart and slightly rotated outward (laterally) about 10–15 degrees for greater balance. Knees, hips and elbows are slightly bent (commonly referred to as "softening your joints"), and arms are rotated slightly forward at the shoulders. This position should have you ready for quick action or reaction in any direction, primarily a median or horizontal plane.

Tip: Don't confuse athletic position with the "ready position" of some sports. For example, a shortstop will have a far deeper knee bend and hip drop to allow for a more explosive lateral or vertical movement when the ball is hit.

Flexion & Extension: Often confused, these are relatively easy to remember once you get the general mental picture. Flexion is accomplished by bending a hinge (elbow, knee) joint, while straightening is extension. Forcing one of these joints past straight is considered hyperextension, and commonly responsible for serious injuries. Note the word "general" above—you can also extend and flex at the hip and shoulder (ball and socket) joints without bending; raising your arm or leg forward and upward is flexion, while returning it to anatomical position is extension. The neck, wrists, fingers and toes all get in on the flexion and extension action, but you get the general idea and you're not getting quizzed.

Rotation: You'll be using this one quite a bit, primarily when twisting the trunk. Simply put, this rotation is bringing the side of the body bisected by the frontal plane toward the medial plane while traveling along the transverse plane. Sorry, couldn't resist. In other words, rotating your trunk so one of your shoulders is aligned with your belly button. Easy, right?

Abduction & Adduction: We don't cover this much in the exercises, but this section would be lacking if we didn't briefly cover these opposite motions. Abduction of the hip or shoulder joint occurs when the leg or arm is lifted outward (laterally) from anatomical position; your shoulder has a much wider range of motion (ROM) and adduction encompasses the entire lateral movement upward of your arm from your side to directly over your head. Adduction is the motion of bringing the arm or leg back to anatomical position. I use a little mnemonic to differentiate between the two: "Abby opens."

Range of Motion (ROM): This is the entire spectrum of movement allowed by one's anatomy and physiology; limits are based on joint, muscle, ligament and cartilage positioning, size, shape and condition—essentially the mechanical limit you could possibly move if you were in top condition. Training to strengthen your musculature and develop more flexibility will allow your joints to function with as wide a ROM as possible. While range of motion basically covers hyperflexion, hyperextension, etc., those conditions are not considered optimal. Therefore, when a trainer (ahem, like me) uses the phrase "complete the movement with as full a range of motion as

possible," this doesn't include putting your joints in a hyper-anything position.

Once you begin the Basic or Advanced *Medicine Ball Workouts* program, perform it at your own pace and within your personal level of fitness. If you're new to working out, especially balance-based training, or returning to exercise after some time off, be sure to take your time and take it easy for the first two weeks to allow your muscles to adjust to the new workload and reduce post-workout soreness. DOMS is the acronym for "delayed onset muscle soreness" and the simple reality is that the soreness you experience 24, 48 or more hours after pushing a workout too hard will hamper, limit or completely sabotage your program. You have plenty of time to get in the groove with this program, so take your time and work your way into it!

This may come as a shock, but no one's perfect at every exercise when they get started—usually far from it! Even after some practice, you still won't be a pro at every movement. Some exercises may come naturally while others feel completely foreign, and almost all unbalanced exercises take a long time to master. Multi-joint, multi-muscle movements like squats are already complicated and difficult to master with just your bodyweight; when you perform them with a weighted medicine ball, they're a much more demanding yet rewarding exercise. It's extremely important to keep working on perfecting the form and get stronger along the way. Don't give up and sit out an exercise if you can't do it—make the investment in yourself and learn the proper form for each move. You'll only reap the benefits.

If you feel extremely fatigued or have an uncomfortable level of pain and soreness, take two to three days off from the workout. Some muscle fatigue and soreness is to be expected and you can continue to exercise carefully when you're a little tired or sore. Any sharp pain, pinches or throbbing aches in your joints is not to be ignored. If the discomfort or pain persists, seek the advice of a medical professional. If you feel any sensation in a joint or muscle that makes you say "uh-oh," then stop immediately, rest and assess whether or not it's a serious injury that needs medical attention.

Due to the nature of a full-body, weighted workout routine, you'll be lifting, pushing and pressing your entire bodyweight along with 4 to 20 additional pounds in your hands. It's very important that you focus on proper form and utilize the proper muscles to complete each exercise. This means no cheating by arching your back on push-ups or allowing your knees to bow in during squats—you're only cheating yourself. Every proper-form rep just gets you closer to your goals!

If you have a pre-existing condition like joint instability or a muscular imbalance, make sure you recognize any physical limitations, take your time and work your way up slowly while focusing on training with good form. It's far more important to be careful with nagging injuries than it is to worry about completing all the exercises in any specified amount of time. Performing the exercises with proper form will help you to

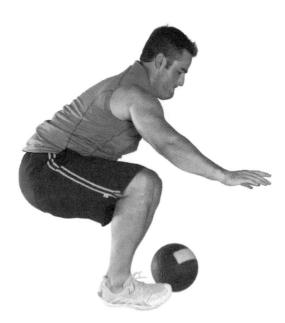

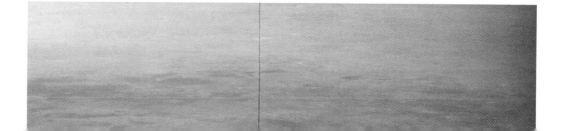

build strength, flexibility and balance as well as improve your sports performance—but not if you ignore the warning signs and hurt yourself. If pain or soreness persists, please see a medical professional.

When performing any exercise routine that requires you to lift, pull or press your bodyweight, don't take any chances with unsafe equipment. In addition, make sure you're properly trained to use any equipment before you start a workout. Always be aware of your surroundings and make sure you have plenty of room to execute moves safely without hitting or tripping over other objects.

Exercise Progression

Guess what, you're not a professional athlete. How do I know? Because you're reading this section. Seriously, every professional athlete I've ever worked with would already be three exercises into the Advanced program—it's just how they're wired. The good news is that, because you're not getting paid to train and perform, you can take your time getting in tune with the workouts and preparing your body to perform each exercise with proper form. No one will be holding a finish line at the end of each workout, and no one will be judging you as you progress from simple to advanced movements. If they're secretly taking inventory of your exercises, then they should focus on their own workout!

Because we're adding weights in the form of a medicine ball to some relatively complicated bodyweight exercises, it's important that you learn and perfect the proper form first before you pick up any weight. If you're not familiar with the exercises, perform as many sets, days or weeks as you need before starting to use the medicine ball. Heck, if you complete an entire program without ever touching a ball, that's still a rousing success! The main goal is finding a routine that you can stick with and developing good fitness habits to support a healthy, active lifestyle. You have plenty of time to progress to the more challenging exercises with weights.

Level 1: Begin with and master each exercise using your bodyweight only.

Level 2: Add light weights that allow you to keep proper form throughout the entire range of motion. Add additional weight as you progress in strength and comfort with the movements.

Level 3: Focus on the specific goals from the chart on page 35: weight loss, toning, muscle gain, endurance, speed. Progress to heavier weights for the muscle building workouts only when you can complete all the desired reps with proper form.

Level 4: Once you've mastered the exercises and techniques and are familiar with the entire program (usually after you've finished the Basic or Advanced programs), start over and perform the workout with the goal of enhanced athletic performance.

Depending on athletic ability, previous workout experience, strength and coordination, some individuals can progress through all of these four levels in the course of a seven-week regimen. Many individuals will need to work through an entire program for each level and that's no problem at all. There's no rush to complete each

of the goals. The workouts in this book—from the Basic to Advanced—are designed to be used as often as you want, for as long as you want, to develop and maintain your fitness and physique. It's up to you to find a balance and a level that work for you, and progress as you're able.

Warming Up & Stretching

Properly warming up the body prior to any activity is very important, as is stretching post-workout. Please note that warming up and stretching are two completely different things: A warm-up routine should be done before stretching so that your muscles are more pliable and able to be stretched efficiently. You should not "warm up" by stretching; you simply don't want to push, pull or stretch cold muscles.

Prior to warming up, your muscles are significantly less flexible. Think of pulling a rubber band out of a freezer: If you stretch it forcefully before it has a chance to warm up, you'll likely tear it. Stretching cold muscles can cause a significantly higher rate of muscle strains and even injuries to joints that rely on those muscles for alignment.

It's crucial to raise your body temperature prior to beginning a workout. In order to prevent injury, such as a muscle strain, you want to loosen up your muscles and joints before you begin the actual exercise movement. A good warm-up before your workout should slowly raise your core body temperature, heart rate and breathing. Before jumping into the workout, you must increase blood flow to all working areas of the body. This augmented blood flow will transport more oxygen and nutrients to the muscles being worked. The warm-up will also increase the range of motion of your joints.

Stretching should generally be done after a workout. It'll help you reduce muscle soreness from the workout, increase range of motion and flexibility within a joint or muscle, and prepare your body for any future workouts. Stretching immediately post-exercise while your muscles are still warm allows your muscles to return to their full range of motion (which gives you more flexibility gains) and reduces the chance of injury or fatigue in the hours or days after an intense workout. It's important to remember that even when you're warm and loose, you should never "bounce" during stretching. Keep your movements slow and controlled.

Here's the proper workout progression to keep in mind:

1. Basic warm-up: Walk, jog, jumping jacks—raise your heart rate and body temperature slightly, loosen up stiff muscles and get a very light sweat (if any).

2. Dynamic warm-up/shake-out: After at least 5 minutes of warm-up, shake out your arms and legs and perform some of the dynamic warm-ups listed on page 104.

3. Perform some slow, controlled bodyweight exercises: Focusing on maintaining perfect form, perform 3–6 bodyweight reps of a multi-joint, multi-muscle exercise like wood chops (page 57) or burpees (page 60). Skip the medicine ball for this warm-up.

4. Work out: Be mindful of your form on every rep. Maintain your intensity and crush your workout.

5. Shake-out/stretch: Shake out your tight muscles, then perform some techniques starting on page 104.

6. Eat: Immediately post-workout, consume a recovery drink with a 4:1 ratio of carbs to protein in order to replenish your glycogen stores and also give your muscles the amino acids they need to repair and strengthen. A protein shake with a banana or chocolate milk are very good choices.

7. Rest: Jump-start the building process by resting. A 20-minute nap after eating never hurts.

Avoiding Injuries

As we covered earlier in the FAQs (page 19), bodyweight strength training combined with weights is an incredibly efficient way to build strength, flexibility and balance as well as develop a lean, ripped physique. Let's be honest, though; none of us are perfect. Due to years of improper posture, sports injuries or even weak musculature, we all have imbalances that can affect proper form and even put us on the fast track to injury. In addition, jumping into a new exercise routine too quickly or doing the exercises with improper form can exacerbate any pre-existing injury. Unstable surfaces make it even more precarious for first-timers or those coming back after a layoff. This is why I recommend starting out by performing bodyweight versions of each exercise before stepping it up by adding in weights.

Throughout the routine, you should expect to experience mild soreness and fatigue, especially when you're just getting started. The feeling of your muscles being "pumped" and the fatigue of an exhausting workout should be expected. These are positive feelings.

On the other hand, any sharp pain, muscle spasm or numbness is a warning sign that you need to stop and not push yourself any harder. Some small muscle groups may fatigue more quickly because they're often overlooked in other workouts. Your hands and forearms are doing a tremendous amount of work and can easily tire out. If you feel you can't grip or support yourself with your hands anymore, take a rest. It's far better than slipping and getting hurt.

Here are a few other symptoms to watch for: sore elbows, shoulder (rotator cuff) pain and stiff neck. Sore elbows are usually a sign that you're locking out your elbows when your arms are fully extended; remember to keep a slight bend in your elbows. Pain in the rotator cuff can be caused by poor form or a hand position that's too wide while doing push-ups or overhead presses.

A stiff neck can result from straining your neck throughout the movement; try to keep your neck loose and flexible. If any of these pains persists, it's imperative that you seek medical advice. Be smart, stay safe and take your time adjusting to the program!

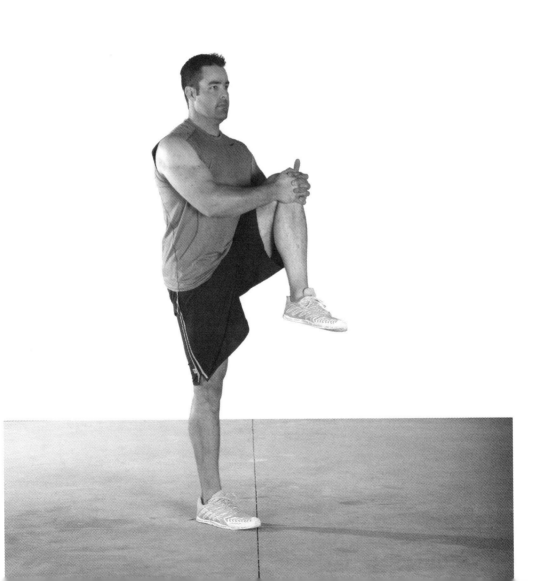

What's Your Motivation?

Let's face it—some days we all feel like we need a good reason just to get out of bed in the morning. I have a great gig writing books and training some awesome folks, but there are plenty of times when I'd like to smash the alarm and bury my head under the covers. Workouts are the same way for most people—if you can think of any reason to skip it, you probably will. I'll admit to missing my share of workouts, but it never seems to be worth it: When I skip one, I just ending up paying for it later with a subpar performance at a race or even feeling miserable because I feel like I've let myself down. Usually the penalty is worse and lasts longer than the workout would've anyway. My wife can always tell when I'm cranky and has even thrown me out of the house to go for a run and cheer-up—and it actually works!

Ninety-nine percent of the time, we feel like superheroes after a good workout. Our endorphins are all cranked and we feel absolutely bulletproof. If we could bottle that experience we'd be millionaires...but more importantly, if we just remind ourselves how great we'll feel when we're done with the training, it makes it that much easier to get psyched up for it. The remaining one percent of the time we either forgot our gym shoes or something. It happens to all of us.

Often misattributed to Beethoven, Ignacy Paderewski mused, "If I miss one day of practice, I notice it. If I miss two days, the critics notice it. If I miss three days, the audience notices it." Fitness is similar yet not exactly the same as a world-renowned musician skipping out on hours of playing scales. We all miss workouts, that's a given; the goal is to find your motivation and make it to far more than you miss.

The bottom line with motivation is that you'll never get through any life change without it. You need to be motivated to change jobs, try a new restaurant, even brush your teeth. Some motivation is easier (and smellier) than others, but every modification to your course of action requires you have the incentive to give it a shot and the follow-through to stick with it.

Here I introduce what I like to refer to as my "ass-ivation" scale, progressive levels of motivation from getting active through developing athletic performance:

GET OFF YOUR ASS-IVATION: This is the most common motivation with individuals as they become more sedentary. It will usually involve an epiphany after finishing off a bag of chips on the couch or just not fitting into your favorite jeans anymore. No matter what Mick Jagger sang back in 1964, time is not on our side, and every day, month or year you spend inactive you're gaining weight, losing athletic ability, stamina and cardiovascular fitness and letting your body go to pot.

LOSE MY ASS-IVATION: This is weight loss and toning, usually for a life event like a wedding, beach vacation, class reunion or newfound single status that forces you to look somewhat presentable to others. "Boot camps" are really popular with this group because they're usually looking for immediate results.

KICK SOME ASS-IVATION: This involves athletic improvement or sport-specific training for an upcoming season or event. Speed, core strength, endurance and flexibility are a common focus for most sports that involve getting from point A to point B as rapidly as possible, especially athletic endeavors where you repeat that over and over (e.g., soccer, football, baseball, paintball, etc.).

Now, these top-three "ass-ivation" goals aren't mutually exclusive. You can lose weight, get healthy, improve your athletic ability and develop a fantastic physique all at the same time. Heck, that's what the programs in this book were created for! Using the "Setting Your Goals" section below, you can begin your preparation and kick your plan into gear by using the Basic or Advanced programs you'll find starting on page 39.

Setting Your Goals

The easiest way to fail at any endeavor is to start without a plan. Sure, you might have a fun time taking a drive without a map (or GPS, smartphone, etc.), but you're going to end up lost, waste a lot of time and never make it to your destination in time! Developing your body is a lot like building a house: Both require a plan and need to start with a solid foundation. Here are some fantastic blueprints for the new you to choose from, each with some specific nutrition and exercise advice to help you take full advantage of the programs.

Goal	Requirements
weight loss	Perform each exercise in rapid succession with little or no time in between. This "circuit training" will keep your heart rate elevated for the entire workout and for hours afterward, helping you burn fat. Combine this with a balanced, healthy diet of 45% protein, 30% carbohydrates and 25% fats.
toning	Similar to the weight-loss plan in terms of nutrition and circuit training, toning requires a great deal of focus on form and squeezing every muscle with every rep. It also doesn't hurt to add some additional repetitions to each set to maximize the fat burn and strengthening of lean muscle.
muscle gain	Gaining muscle requires using heavier weights and keeping your muscles under tension for longer periods of time. Slower recovery phases and rapid exertion phases with weighted movements does the trick. Focus on the form of each exercise and perform it with the heaviest weight possible. Move slowly between sets and exercises, taking a 30-second break. Each week, you'll be adding more weight or additional reps to continue to grow your muscles. Also, you'll be adding more protein to your diet—about 1 gram of protein relative to your target body weight. If you're looking to get to 165 pounds, that means you'll be eating upwards of 165 grams of protein a day.
endurance	Less about heavy weights and more about prolonged exertion, building endurance is similar to weight loss (above) and greatly benefitted by adding 2–3 additional sets to your workout. By training your body to keep performing after fatigue, you push the barrier of exhaustion further away. "Going long" requires additional slow-burning carbohydrates for fuel (whole wheat, sweet potatoes, etc.). Approximately 40% protein, 40% carbs and 20% fats is pretty common for endurance athletes looking to stay fueled yet remain as light as possible.
speed	Quick, explosive movements are the name of the game to build speed. You're looking to activate and develop your fast-twitch muscle fibers by performing plyometric movements, combining sprints, explosive tosses and "amping up" exercises. Add moves like squat jumps, burpees or mountain climbers (these and more descriptions and photos are available at www.7weekstofitness.com) to your workouts and perform each exercise with high intensity. Fueling and nutrition is similar to weight loss but with just a little more carbohydrates for refueling after a hard workout; shoot for 40–45% protein, 35–40% carbs and the remaining 15–25% healthy fats.
enhanced athletic performance	A well-rounded program contains elements of weight loss, toning, muscle gain, endurance and speed spread out throughout the course of a week's workouts, switching it up each week. For example, Monday = toning & endurance, Wednesday = speed & weight loss, Friday = muscle gain. Nutrition needs are based on the specific goals: lower carbs for weight loss, more protein for muscle gain or more carbs for replenishment after speed or endurance workouts.

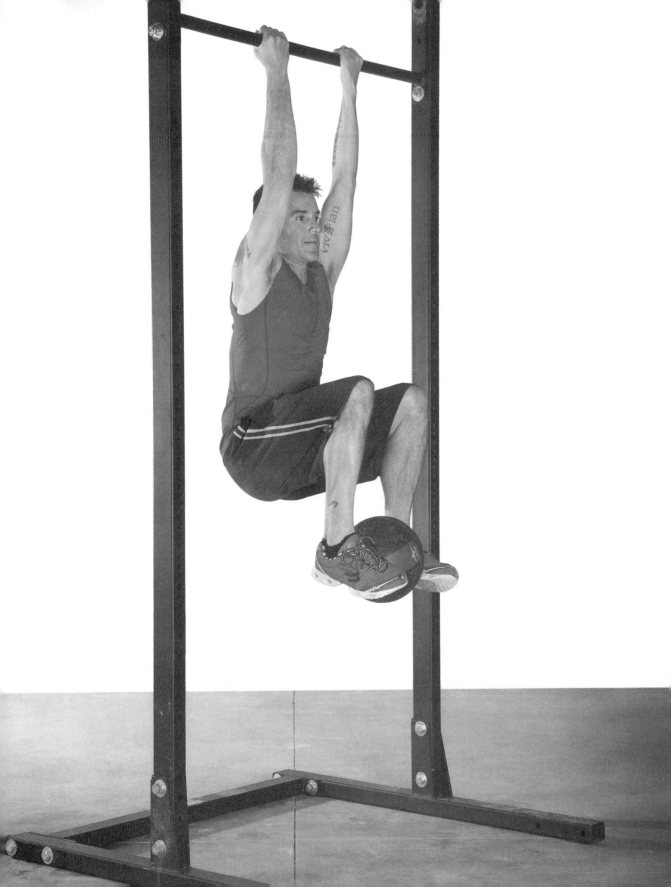

PART 2: PROGRAMS

Like I mentioned earlier in "Preparing for the Workouts" (page 25), you're not a pro and no one expects you to be—especially me! Right from the start, it's important that you learn the proper form and full range of motion of each exercise in addition to assessing your physical limits. The quickest way to get knocked off track in your workouts is to do too much too soon. Too many reps, weights that are too heavy, or not enough rest and recovery between workouts are common culprits. Squats and lunges are exercises that are quite common for producing soreness and fatigue the day or two following a strenuous workout, so take it easy through the first week or as long as you need to get on track and comfortable with the workload.

Remember, there's no finish line or anyone waiting at the end of the programs to hand you an award—the reward is simply being fit, healthy and feeling great. The finish line also isn't just one spot; you'll catch glimpses of it every time you look in the mirror and with every compliment you receive. To give credit to the great marketing slogan used by Nike: "There is no finish line." There truly isn't. You can always continue to improve, but make sure to enjoy yourself along the way!

In the following pages, you'll find the Basic and Advanced programs. Both are based on a lot of the same exercises, with the Advanced program building on the solid foundation of the Basic program. If you haven't worked out pretty regularly following a full-body functional cross-training routine like P90X, Insanity or CrossFit, I recommend you start with the Basic program to assess your fitness level and get used to performing each exercise with proper form. You can always progress up to the Advanced program when you're ready.

A WORD ABOUT INTENSITY

The workouts in this book are relatively straightforward and can be performed by most athletic individuals, but to get the most out of this and any exercise program, it's all about performing the moves and routines with the maximum intensity you can muster. Once you've learned how to perform the exercises with proper technique and build a base of fitness and endurance, you should continue to push yourself from workout to workout. You may not reach this threshold for weeks or even after completing one or both of the programs, and that's totally cool. The important part is that when you're ready to push yourself and increase the intensity, speed or weight, you do so. To continue to improve your performance, you need to continue to improve your workouts; add some sprints to the beginning or an additional set at the end, pick up a heavier medicine ball and set your goals on tossing it farther than you have before or, my favorite, use a timer for your workouts and progress through each one faster than the last. It's up to you to push your limits to get progressively better results. I can't be there motivating you for each workout so you need to stoke those fires yourself!

Basic Program

Welcome to the start of a new you! Right now, you're on the ground level and are about to start building a foundation of fitness through strength-building bodyweight exercises and the addition of medicine balls and more explosive movements once you're ready. This progressive program is a great starting point for nearly all but the most conditioned athletes, because you can focus on nailing your form and prepping your mind and body for progressively harder workouts to come.

As I mentioned at least a couple times so far, take it at your own pace. Start with bodyweight versions, then add the medicine ball as you're ready. The chart below progresses through the same three-day-per-week exercise routine for four weeks, increasing in repetitions. Since you'll be choosing your own medicine ball, you can increase the weight as you see fit and are able to perform each exercise with flawless form.

I recommend starting without a ball until you master the movements, then progress to using a light one and so on. This program can be repeated as many times as you feel necessary. Just remember: If you're interested in seeing fitness gains, you'll continually need to raise reps or medicine ball weight from week to week.

COMMENTS

- Take as little rest as needed between exercises, and a 2-minute break between sets.
- Take at least one day of rest in between workouts (Monday, Wednesday and Friday work very well), and make sure you stay active on the weekend. Play some of the games (page 97), perhaps?

Note: Based on the goals on page 35, modify your rest between exercises and sets as well as your number of sets accordingly.

- During this progression, you may increase the weight of your medicine ball(s) if you choose, provided you can still complete all the repetitions with proper form.
- You may also choose to complete the entire Basic program without a medicine ball (replace wall ball with ball thruster) and then repeat the entire program with a light ball, progressing to heavier weights on subsequent workouts.

Week 1		Rest 2 minutes after every set			
Mon set 1	3 Goblet Squats page 54	6 Mason Twists page 73	6 Good Mornings page 74	4 Push-Ups page 70	:25 Plank page 66
set 2	3 Ball Thrusters page 55	4 Elephant Twists page 65	5 Sit-Ups page 76	4 Curl & Presses (per arm) page 71	6 Crunch w/Toe Touches page 77
set 3	5 Romanian Deadlifts page 59	6 T-Twists page 64	4 Supermans page 75	6 Press & Triceps Ext. page 72	6 Mason Twists page 73
Tues		Rest			
Wed set 1	3 Ball Thrusters page 55	4 Lunge & Twists page 58	4 Supermans page 75	5 Sit-Ups page 76	6 Press & Triceps Ext. page 72
set 2	5 Wall Balls page 56	5 Romanian Deadlifts page 59	6 Good Mornings page 74	:25 Plank page 66	4 Curl & Presses (per arm) page 71
set 3	4 Wood Chops page 57	3 Goblet Squats page 54	6 Mason Twists page 73	6 Crunch w/Toe Touches page 77	4 Push-Ups page 70
Thur		Rest			
Fri set 1	4 Wood Chops page 57	3 Ball Thrusters page 55	5 Sit-Ups page 76	6 T-Twists page 64	4 Push-Ups page 70
set 2	6 Mason Twists page 73	5 Romanian Deadlifts page 59	:25 Plank page 66	4 Supermans page 75	4 Curl & Presses (per arm) page 71
set 3	5 Wall Balls page 56	4 Lunge & Twists page 58	6 Crunch w/Toe Touches page 77	6 Good Mornings page 74	6 Press & Triceps Ext. page 72

Week 2

Rest 2 minutes after every set

Mon set 1	5 Goblet Squats page 54	8 Mason Twists page 73	8 Good Mornings page 74	6 Push-Ups page 70	:35 Plank page 66
set 2	5 Ball Thrusters page 55	6 Elephant Twists page 65	7 Sit-Ups page 76	6 Curl & Presses (per arm) page 71	8 Crunch w/Toe Touches page 77
set 3	7 Romanian Deadlifts page 59	8 T-Twists page 64	6 Supermans page 75	8 Press & Triceps Ext. page 72	8 Mason Twists page 73
Tues			Rest		
Wed set 1	5 Ball Thrusters page 55	6 Lunge & Twists page 58	6 Supermans page 75	7 Sit-Ups page 76	8 Press & Triceps Ext. page 72
set 2	7 Wall Balls page 56	7 Romanian Deadlifts page 59	8 Good Mornings page 74	:35 Plank page 66	6 Curl & Presses (per arm) page 71
set 3	6 Wood Chops page 57	5 Goblet Squats page 54	8 Mason Twists page 73	8 Crunch w/Toe Touches page 77	6 Push-Ups page 70
Thur			Rest		
Fri set 1	6 Wood Chops page 57	6 Ball Thrusters page 55	7 Sit-Ups page 76	8 T- Twists	6 Push-Ups page 70
set 2	8 Mason Twists page 73	7 Romanian Deadlifts page 59	:35 Plank page 66	6 Supermans page 75	6 Curl & Presses (per arm) page 71
set 3	7 Wall Balls page 56	6 Lunge & Twists page 58	8 Crunch w/Toe Touches page 77	8 Good Mornings page 74	8 Press & Triceps Ext. page 72

Week 3		Rest 2 minutes after every set			
Mon set 1	7 Goblet Squats page 54	10 Mason Twists page 73	10 Good Mornings page 74	8 Push-Ups page 70	:45 Plank page 66
set 2	7 Ball Thrusters page 55	8 Elephant Twists page 65	9 Sit-Ups page 76	8 Curl & Presses (per arm) page 71	10 Crunch w/Toe Touches page 77
set 3	9 Romanian Deadlifts page 59	10 T-Twists page 64	8 Supermans page 75	10 Press & Triceps Ext. page 72	10 Mason Twists page 73
Tues		Rest			
Wed set 1	7 Ball Thrusters page 55	8 Lunge & Twists page 58	8 Supermans page 75	9 Sit-Ups page 76	10 Press & Triceps Ext. page 72
set 2	9 Wall Balls page 56	9 Romanian Deadlifts page 59	10 Good Mornings page 74	:45 Plank page 66	8 Curl & Presses (per arm) page 71
set 3	8 Wood Chops page 57	7 Goblet Squats page 54	10 Mason Twists page 73	10 Crunch w/Toe Touches page 77	8 Push-Ups page 70
Thur		Rest			
Fri set 1	8 Wood Chops page 57	8 Ball Thrusters page 55	9 Sit-Ups page 76	10 T- Twists page 64	8 Push-Ups page 70
set 2	10 Mason Twists page 73	9 Romanian Deadlifts page 59	:45 Plank page 66	8 Supermans page 75	8 Curl & Presses (per arm) page 71
set 3	9 Wall Balls page 56	8 Lunge & Twists page 58	10 Crunch w/Toe Touches page 77	10 Good Mornings page 74	10 Press & Triceps Ext. page 72

Week 4 — Rest 2 minutes after every set

Mon	set 1	9 Goblet Squats *page 54*	12 Mason Twists *page 73*	12 Good Mornings *page 74*	10 Push-Ups *page 70*	1:05 Plank *page 66*
	set 2	9 Ball Thrusters *page 55*	10 Elephant Twists *page 65*	11 Sit-Ups *page 76*	10 Curl & Presses (per arm) *page 71*	12 Crunch w/Toe Touches *page 77*
	set 3	11 Romanian Deadlifts *page 59*	12 T-Twists *page 64*	10 Supermans *page 75*	12 Press & Triceps Ext. *page 72*	12 Mason Twists *page 73*
Tues		Rest				
Wed	set 1	9 Ball Thrusters *page 55*	10 Lunge & Twists *page 58*	10 Supermans *page 75*	11 Sit-Ups *page 76*	12 Press & Triceps Ext. *page 72*
	set 2	11 Wall Balls *page 56*	11 Romanian Deadlifts *page 59*	12 Good Mornings *page 74*	1:05 Plank *page 66*	10 Curl & Presses (per arm) *page 71*
	set 3	10 Wood Chops *page 57*	9 Goblet Squats *page 54*	12 Mason Twists *page 73*	12 Crunch w/Toe Touches *page 77*	10 Push-Ups *page 70*
Thur		Rest				
Fri	set 1	10 Wood Chops *page 57*	10 Ball Thrusters *page 55*	11 Sit-Ups *page 76*	12 T-Twists *page 64*	10 Push-Ups *page 70*
	set 2	12 Mason Twists *page 73*	11 Romanian Deadlifts *page 59*	1:05 Plank *page 66*	10 Supermans *page 75*	10 Curl & Presses (per arm) *page 71*
	set 3	11 Wall Balls *page 56*	10 Lunge & Twists *page 58*	12 Crunch w/Toe Touches *page 77*	12 Good Mornings *page 74*	12 Press & Triceps Ext. *page 72*

Advanced Program

Congratulations on reaching the Advanced program! I hope you enjoyed progressing through the Basic program to get here and learned a lot about the exercises (and yourself) along the way. If you're jumping straight into the Advanced program, you should be extremely familiar with performing each of the exercises in the upcoming charts with flawless form and be adept at using the medicine ball to make these exercises more strenuous and effective. If that doesn't sound like your level of fitness, there's no shame at all in starting with the Basic program to learn the ropes and build a rock-solid foundation for fitness.

Like the Basic program, this routine gets progressively more difficult. The differentiator between the two is the additional tosses, sprints and some advanced movements on the fourth day of the program. I also strongly recommend upping the intensity (see "A Word about Intensity" on page 38) and making each workout count. Completing this program should be difficult yet achievable, and by the end you should feel proud of your accomplishment. If not, most likely you didn't push the intensity as much as you could've.

The chart below progresses through the same four-day-per-week exercise routine for four weeks, increasing in repetitions. Since you'll be choosing your own medicine ball, you can increase the weight as you see fit and are able to perform each exercise with flawless form. This program can be repeated as many times as you feel necessary, just remember if you're interested in seeing fitness gains, you'll continually need to raise reps or medicine ball weight from week to week.

COMMENTS

- Take as little rest as needed between exercises, and a 1-minute break between sets.
- During this progression, you may increase the weight of your medicine ball(s) if you choose, provided you can still complete all the repetitions with proper form.

Note: Based on the goals on page 35, modify your rest between exercises and sets as well as your number of sets accordingly.

Week 1

Week 1		Rest 1 minute after every set				
Mon	*set 1*	10 Wood Chops *page 57*	12 Mason Twists *page 73*	12 Crunch w/Toe Touches *page 77*	12 Wall Balls *page 56*	10 Push-Ups *page 70*
	set 2	10 Lunge & Twists *page 58*	12 T-Twists *page 64*	10 Sit-Ups *page 76*	12 Ball Thrusters *page 55*	8 T Push-Ups *page 69*
	set 3	12 Romanian Deadlifts *page 59*	10 Elephant Twists *page 65*	1:00 Plank *page 66*	6 Burpees *page 60*	10 2-Hand Push-Up *page 70*
Tues		Rest				
Wed	*set 1*	6 Burpees *page 60*	10 Supermans *page 75*	10 Lunge & Twists *page 58*	10 Sit-Ups *page 76*	12 Curl & Presses (per arm) *page 71*
	set 2	4 Turkish Get-Ups *page 79*	12 Good Mornings *page 74*	12 Romanian Deadlifts *page 59*	12 Crunch w/Toe Touches *page 77*	12 Press & Triceps Ext. *page 72*
	set 3	6 Bizarro Burpees *page 62*	10 Supermans *page 75*	10 Wood Chops *page 57*	4 Roll-Outs *page 67*	10 Push-Ups *page 70*
Thur		Rest				
Fri	*set 1*	12 Wall Balls *page 56*	12 Romanian Deadlifts *page 59*	4 Roll-Outs *page 67*	12 Press & Triceps Ext. *page 72*	12 Good Mornings *page 74*
	set 2	12 Ball Thrusters *page 55*	10 Wood Chops *page 57*	1:00 Plank *page 66*	10 2-Hand Push-Ups *page 70*	10 Supermans *page 75*
	set 3	10 Lunge & Twists *page 58*	:30 Figure 8 *page 78*	12 Crunch w/Toe Touches *page 77*	12 Curl & Presses (per arm) *page 71*	12 Push-Ups *page 70*
Sat	*set 1*	12 Wall Balls *page 56*	10 Lunge & Twists *page 58*	3:00 Toss & Run *page 98*	Rest :30	6 Burpees *page 60*
	set 2	12 Ball Thrusters *page 55*	12 Romanian Deadlifts *page 59*	3:00 Out & Back Sprints *page 98*	Rest :30	4 Turkish Get-Ups *page 79*
	set 3	10 Wood Chops *page 57*	12 Goblet Squats *page 54*	18 Distance Tosses *page 98*	Rest :30	6 Bizarro Burpees *page 62*

Week 2

Rest 1 minute after every set

Mon	set 1	13 Wood Chops page 57	15 Mason Twists page 73	15 Crunch w/Toe Touches page 77	15 Wall Balls page 56	13 Push-Ups page 70
	set 2	13 Lunge & Twists page 58	15 T-Twists page 64	13 Sit-Ups page 76	15 Ball Thrusters page 55	11 T Push-Ups page 69
	set 3	8 Romanian Deadlifts page 58	9 Elephant Twists page 65	7 Supermans page 75	9 Press & Triceps Ext. page 72	9 Mason Twists page 73
Tues				Rest		
Wed	set 1	9 Burpees page 60	13 Supermans page 75	13 Lunge & Twists page 58	13 Sit-Ups page 76	15 Curl & Presses (per arm) page 71
	set 2	6 Turkish Get-Ups page 79	15 Good Mornings page 74	15 Romanian Deadlifts page 59	15 Crunch w/Toe Touches page 77	15 Press & Triceps Ext. page 72
	set 3	9 Bizarro Burpees page 62	13 Supermans page 75	13 Wood Chops page 57	7 Roll-Outs page 67	13 Push-Ups page 70
Thur				Rest		
Fri	set 1	15 Wall Balls page 56	15 Romanian Deadlifts page 59	7 Roll-Outs page 67	15 Press & Triceps Ext. page 72	15 Good Mornings page 74
	set 2	15 Ball Thrusters page 55	13 Wood Chops page 57	1:20 Plank page 66	13 2-Hand Push-Up page 70	13 Supermans page 75
	set 3	13 Lunge & Twists page 58	:50 Figure 8 page 78	15 Crunch w/Toe Touches page 77	15 Curl & Presses (per arm) page 71	15 Push-Ups page 70
Sat	set 1	15 Wall Balls page 56	13 Lunge & Twists page 58	3:20 Toss & Run page 98	Rest :30	9 Burpees page 60
	set 2	15 Ball Thrusters page 55	15 Romanian Deadlifts page 59	3:20 Out & Back Sprints page 98	Rest :30	6 Turkish Get-Ups page 79
	set 3	13 Wood Chops page 57	15 Goblet Squats page 54	21 Distance Tosses page 98	Rest :30	9 Bizarro Burpees page 62

Week 3

Rest 1 minute after every set

Mon	set 1	16 Wood Chops *page 57*	18 Mason Twists *page 73*	18 Crunch w/Toe Touches *page 77*	18 Wall Balls *page 56*	16 Push-Ups *page 70*
	set 2	16 Lunge & Twists *page 58*	18 T-Twists *page 64*	16 Sit-Ups *page 76*	18 Ball Thrusters *page 55*	14 T Push-Ups *page 69*
	set 3	11 Romanian Deadlifts *page 58*	12 Elephant Twists *page 65*	10 Supermans *page 75*	12 Press & Triceps Ext. *page 72*	12 Mason Twists *page 73*
Tues		Rest				
Wed	set 1	12 Burpees *page 60*	16 Supermans *page 75*	16 Lunge & Twists *page 58*	16 Sit-Ups *page 76*	18 Curl & Presses (per arm) *page 71*
	set 2	8 Turkish Get-Ups *page 79*	18 Good Mornings *page 74*	18 Romanian Deadlifts *page 59*	18 Crunch w/Toe Touches *page 77*	18 Press & Triceps Ext. *page 72*
	set 3	12 Bizarro Burpees *page 62*	16 Supermans *page 75*	16 Wood Chops *page 57*	10 Roll-Outs *page 67*	16 Push-Ups *page 70*
Thur		Rest				
Fri	set 1	18 Wall Balls *page 56*	18 Romanian Deadlifts *page 59*	10 Roll-Outs *page 67*	18 Press & Triceps Ext. *page 72*	18 Good Mornings *page 74*
	set 2	18 Ball Thrusters *page 55*	16 Wood Chops *page 57*	1:40 Plank *page 66*	16 2-Hand Push-Ups *page 70*	16 Supermans *page 75*
	set 3	16 Lunge & Twists *page 58*	1:10 Figure 8 *page 78*	18 Crunch w/Toe Touches *page 77*	18 Curl & Presses (per arm) *page 71*	18 Push-Ups *page 70*
Sat	set 1	18 Wall Balls *page 56*	16 Lunge & Twists *page 58*	3:40 Toss & Run *page 98*	Rest :30	12 Burpees *page 60*
	set 2	18 Ball Thrusters *page 55*	18 Romanian Deadlifts *page 59*	3:40 Out & Back Sprints *page 98*	Rest :30	8 Turkish Get-Ups *page 79*
	set 3	16 Wood Chops *page 57*	18 Goblet Squats *page 54*	24 Distance Tosses *page 98*	Rest :30	12 Bizarro Burpees *page 62*

Week 4 — Rest 1 minute after every set

Mon set 1	19 Wood Chops page 57	21 Mason Twists page 73	21 Crunch w/Toe Touches page 77	21 Wall Balls page 56	19 Push-Ups page 70
set 2	19 Lunge & Twists page 58	21 T-Twists page 64	19 Sit-Ups page 76	21 Ball Thrusters page 55	17 T Push-Ups page 69
set 3	14 Romanian Deadlifts page 58	15 Elephant Twists page 65	13 Supermans page 75	15 Press & Triceps Ext. page 72	15 Mason Twists page 73
Tues			Rest		
Wed set 1	15 Burpees page 60	19 Supermans page 75	19 Lunge & Twists page 58	19 Sit-Ups page 76	21 Curl & Presses (per arm) page 71
set 2	10 Turkish Get-Ups page 79	21 Good Mornings page 74	21 Romanian Deadlifts page 59	21 Crunch w/Toe Touches page 77	21 Press & Triceps Ext. page 72
set 3	15 Bizarro Burpees page 62	19 Supermans page 75	19 Wood Chops page 57	13 Roll-Outs page 67	19 Push-Ups page 70
Thur			Rest		
Fri set 1	21 Wall Balls page 56	21 Romanian Deadlifts page 59	13 Roll-Outs page 67	21 Press & Triceps Ext. page 72	21 Good Mornings page 74
set 2	21 Ball Thrusters page 55	19 Wood Chops page 57	2:00 Plank page 66	19 2-Hand Push-Up page 70	19 Supermans page 75
set 3	19 Lunge & Twists page 58	1:30 Figure 8 page 78	21 Crunch w/Toe Touches page 77	21 Curl & Presses (per arm) page 71	21 Push-Ups page 70
Sat set 1	21 Wall Balls page 56	19 Lunge & Twists page 58	4:00 Toss & Run page 98	Rest :30	15 Burpees page 60
set 2	21 Ball Thrusters page 55	21 Romanian Deadlifts page 59	4:00 Out & Back Sprints page 98	Rest :30	10 Turkish Get-Ups page 79
set 3	19 Wood Chops page 57	18 Goblet Squats page 54	27 Distance Tosses page 98	Rest :30	15 Bizarro Burpees page 62

Maintaining Your Physique

Congratulations on completing the Advanced program! I hope it was a fun challenge that you're proud of! I've been extremely lucky to be able to share dozens of different programs and hundreds of exercises, stretches, warm-ups, routines and games so far in my 7 Weeks to Fitness and Ultimate Workouts book series. It's an amazing and humbling experience when I receive e-mails or Facebook posts from around the world thanking me for any of my books making a difference in someone's life. Nearly all of those messages end with the question: "What do I do next?"

So what should you do after you complete these programs? The first thing I recommend to anyone completing the Basic and Advanced programs is to switch up workouts and try something new. All of my books are based around six- to eight-week programs for good reason: Every two months or so you need to vary your workouts to avoid hitting plateaus. Keeping your body exercising on a multitude of different planes, hitting primary, secondary and stabilizing muscles with new moves, and developing functional strength means you can't just stick with one routine. Throughout the year I recommend completing several different ones timed specifically to meet your health and fitness goals. At www.7weekstofitness.com, we feature a growing list of routines taken directly from my books—all for free—that you can try out to help find which ones work for you. You can also find a 50+ page sample of each book to help you make your decision. The full books themselves (ePub, print and even smartphone apps) contain a lot more info about performing each of the exercises, nutritional info, games, tips, tricks and more.

PART 3: EXERCISES

Goblet Squat

If you find your knees rolling inward while doing this move, rotate your toes outward a bit more.

TARGET: Quadriceps femoris (quads), gluteus maximus and minimus (glutes), hamstrings, erector spinae, rectus abdominis (abs)

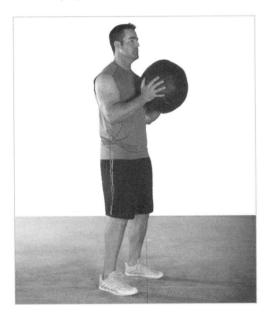

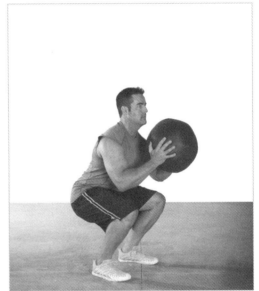

STARTING POSITION: From an athletic position, hold a medicine ball to your chest with your arms bent.

ADVANCED VARIATION: For more quad and glute activation, place another medicine ball on the floor a few inches behind your heels and touch your butt to it at the bottom of your movement.

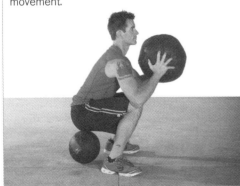

1 Keeping your head up, eyes forward and core tight, bend at the hips and knees and "sit back" just a little, as if you were about to sit directly down into a chair. As you descend, contract your glutes while your body leans forward slightly so that your shoulders are almost in line with your knees. Your knees should not extend past your toes and your weight should remain between the heels and the middle of your feet—don't roll up on the balls of your feet, and don't let your knees roll inward (pronate). Continue the downward motion until your knees are at least 90 degrees and your thighs are parallel to the floor.

Keeping the medicine ball at chest height, push straight up from your heels back to start position. Don't lock your knees at the top of the exercise.

Ball Thruster

TARGET: Quadriceps femoris (quads), gluteus maximus and minimus (glutes), hamstrings, erector spinae, rectus abdominis (abs), deltoids, triceps

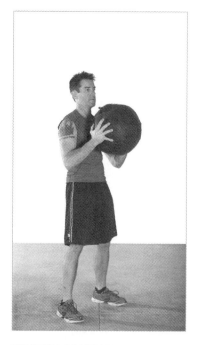 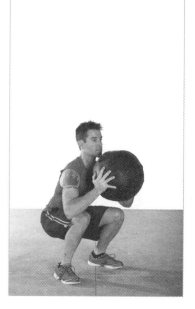 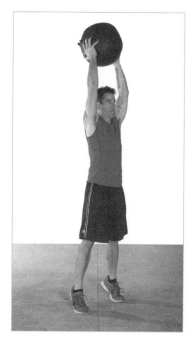

STARTING POSITION: From an athletic position, hold a medicine ball to your chest with your arms bent.

1 Bend at the hips and lower your body into a goblet squat (page 54) until your knees are bent at least 90 degrees. Pause.

2 While pushing straight up from your heels back to standing, press the medicine ball directly overhead by rotating your shoulders forward and extending your arms; your biceps should finish in line with your ears. Don't lock your knees at the top of the exercise. Keep your core flexed throughout the movement and don't arch your back when you lift the ball overhead. Pause.

Carefully reverse the motion and return the ball back to your chest.

Wall Ball

TARGET: Quadriceps femoris (quads), gluteus maximus and minimus (glutes), hamstrings, erector spinae, rectus abdominis (abs), deltoids, triceps, gastrocnemius (calves)

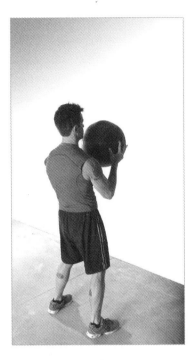 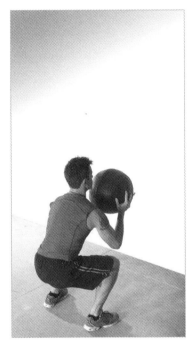 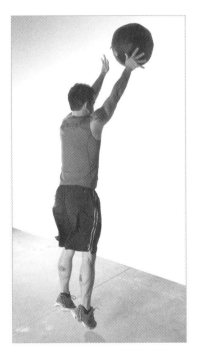

STARTING POSITION: From an athletic position facing a wall about 2 feet away, hold a medicine ball to your chest with your arms bent. Look up and pick a spot on the wall that's at least 8 feet above the floor—that'll be your target to hit with the ball.

1 Bend at the hips and lower your body into a goblet squat (page 54) until your knees are bent at least 90 degrees. Pause.

2 Push straight up from your heels back to standing while explosively pressing and tossing the medicine ball upward and slightly forward to the target on the wall; your biceps should finish in line with your ears. Your weight should transfer to your forefeet as you explode upward, and your feet should leave the ground.

Land with your knees bent, keeping an eye on the ball the entire time. Catch the ball with your elbows bent then carefully return the ball back to your chest, making sure not to bonk yourself in the head, nose or chin.

Wood Chop

TARGET: Quadriceps femoris (quads), gluteus maximus and minimus (glutes), hamstrings, erector spinae, rectus abdominis (abs), deltoids, triceps

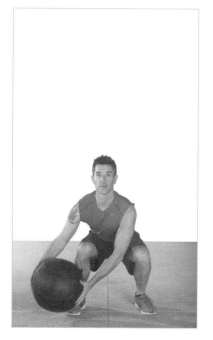 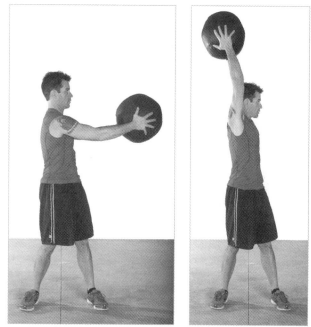

STARTING POSITION: From an athletic position, hold a medicine ball to your chest with your arms bent and initiate a squat (see page 54 for goblet squat technique): Drop your torso straight down until your legs are past parallel; your butt should be as close to the floor as you can get without falling backward. Don't let your knees bow inward, which can cause injury. Slowly bring the ball toward your right foot using your arms; your shoulders and hips should remain pointing straight forward. Don't lean to the right because the imbalance of the weight helps to work your left obliques to maintain proper position.

1–2 Pressing through your heels, raise your torso straight up and lift the ball up and toward the left side of your body. When the ball reaches your left shoulder, twist your core to the left and continue pressing the ball directly overhead, with both arms fully extended, back straight, head up high and looking to the left, and your entire core engaged (abs and glutes contracted) to keep you in a stable position. During the twist and top position, your hips should be pointing forward as much as possible.

Slowly return the ball back to the starting position in a controlled manner. Repeat to the other side. That's 1 rep.

Lunge & Twist

TARGET: Quadriceps femoris (quads), gluteus maximus and minimus (glutes), hamstrings, erector spinae, rectus abdominis (abs), hip flexors, obliques

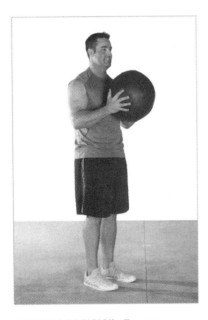

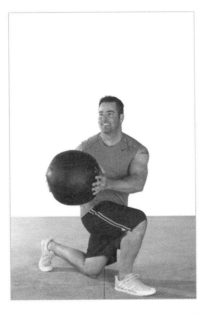

STARTING POSITION: From an athletic position, hold a medicine ball in front of you with your elbows by your sides and your arms bent 90 degrees.

1 Keeping the ball directly in front of you and your core engaged, back straight and head up throughout the exercise, take a large step forward with your right foot, bend both knees and drop your hips straight down until both knees are bent 90 degrees. Your left knee should almost be touching the ground with your left toes on the ground behind you. During the downward motion, twist your core and rotate your torso laterally to your right until both knees are bent 90 degrees and your arms are extended and holding the medicine ball to the right, 90 degrees from where you started. Don't let your forward knee roll inward; your knee should be horizontally in line with your hip on the medial plane and directly above your ankle vertically.

Pushing up through your right heel, straighten both knees and return to starting position.

Repeat to the other side. That's 1 rep.

Romanian Deadlift

TARGET: Gluteus maximus and minimus (glutes), hamstrings, erector spinae

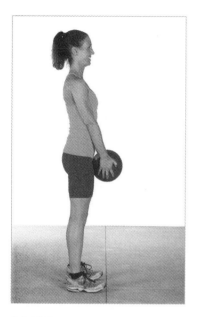 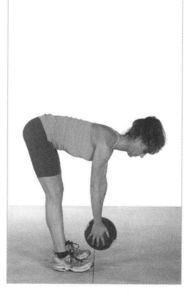 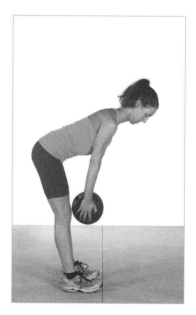

STARTING POSITION: From an athletic position, hold a medicine ball at your waist with your arms fully extended.

1 Keeping your lower back straight and knees slightly bent, bend at the waist to lower the ball as close as you can to your legs as you descend. Don't bounce at the bottom of the movement—descend in a slow, controlled manner and maintain your balance. Keep your shoulders back to prevent your upper back from rounding. Pause.

2 Engage your hamstrings and glutes to assist your lower back in raising your body back to start position.

That's 1 rep.

Burpee

TARGET: Quadriceps femoris (quads), gluteus maximus and minimus (glutes), hamstrings, erector spinae, rectus abdominis (abs), deltoids, forearms, triceps, biceps, gastrocnemius (calves)

STARTING POSITION: From an athletic position, hold a medicine ball to your chest with your arms bent.

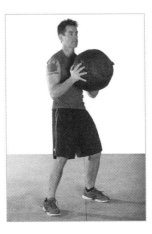

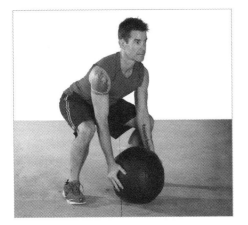

1 Shift your hips backward and "sit back" into a squat (see page 54), keeping your head up and bending your knees. At the bottom of the downward motion, lean your weight forward and place the ball on the floor between your feet, engaging your core, chest, shoulders and arms to create a stable base.

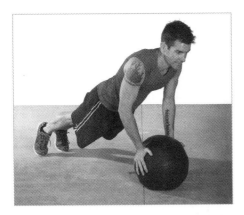

2 Kick your feet straight back so that you're now in a push-up position, forming a nice line from your head to your feet. Keep your core tight to maintain an erect spine.

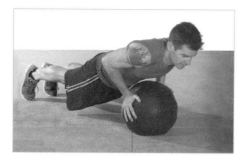

3 Inhale as you lower your torso toward the medicine ball, performing a push-up (page 70). Stop when your body touches the ball.

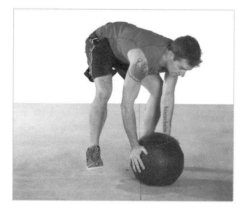

4 Using your chest and arms, press your body up as explosively as possible in order to raise your entire torso, hands and medicine ball off the floor while simultaneously bringing your feet under your body and placing them on the floor underneath your hips.

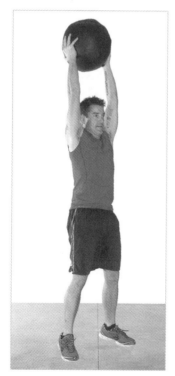

5 Exhale and continue extending the ball directly overhead while pushing off from your forefeet to jump straight up in the air as high as possible.

Land with your knees and elbows slightly bent to absorb the impact before descending into your next rep.

Bizarro Burpee

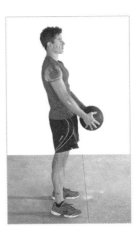

TARGET: Quadriceps femoris (quads), gluteus maximus and minimus (glutes), hamstrings, erector spinae, rectus abdominis (abs), forearms, triceps, biceps, gastrocnemius (calves)

STARTING POSITION: From an athletic position, hold a medicine ball at your waist with your arms extended.

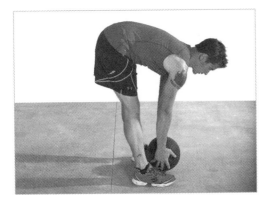

1 Keeping your lower back straight and knees slightly bent, bend at the waist and lower the medicine ball to the ground between your feet, tracking close to your legs the entire way down.

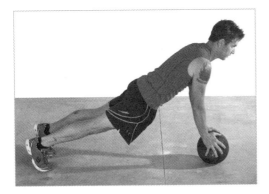

2 Place both hands securely on the top of the medicine ball, squat down and kick your feet out behind you, extending your legs and placing the balls of your feet and toes on the floor for balance. A snapshot of this position should look exactly like a medicine ball plank.

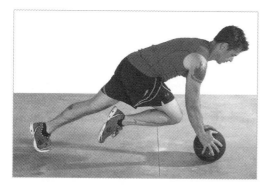

3 With your upper body balanced on the medicine ball, lift your right foot, bend your right knee and pull it up toward your right elbow, stopping before you make contact.

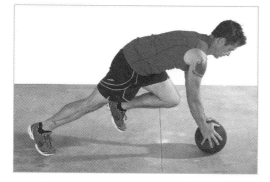

4 Extend your right knee and place your foot back on the floor. Now bring your left knee to your left elbow.

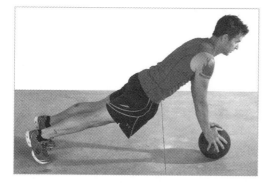

5 Extend your left leg back.

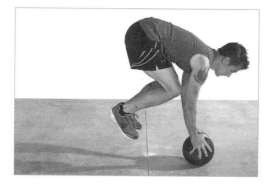

6 Bending at the waist, hop both feet back on each side of the medicine ball, straighten your legs and lift the medicine ball back to start position, engaging your hamstrings and glutes to assist your lower back to extend your waist.

T-Twist

TARGET: Erector spinae, rectus abdominis (abs), obliques, forearms, triceps

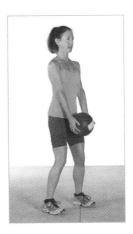

STARTING POSITION: From an athletic position, hold a medicine ball at your waist with your arms extended.

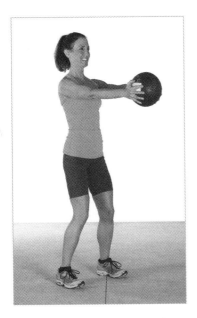

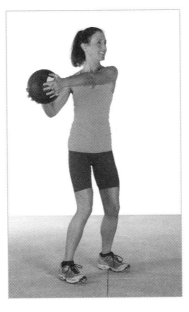

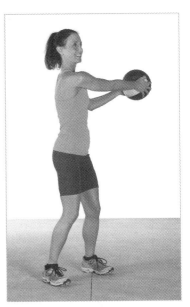

1 Keeping your core tight and back straight, raise the medicine ball to shoulder height, directly in front of your torso with arms fully extended. Pause.

2 With your knees slightly bent, keep your hips facing forward while using your oblique muscles to rotate your upper body and the ball 90 degrees (or as far as you can go) to the right.

3 Slowly return to start position. Pause, then repeat to the other side.

That's 1 rep.

Elephant Twist

Start without a medicine ball or use a very light one until you get comfortable with this exercise, and never bounce or swing during the movement.

TARGET: Gluteus maximus and minimus (glutes), hamstrings, erector spinae, obliques

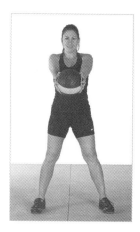

STARTING POSITION: From an athletic position, hold a medicine ball in front of you with your arms extended.

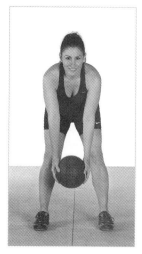

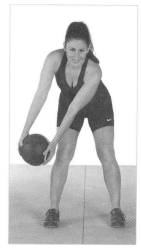

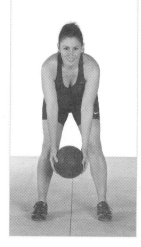

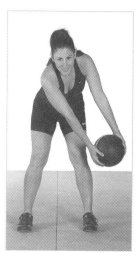

1 Bend forward at the waist 90 degrees so that the ball is hanging from your arms just above your feet.

2 Using your core, slowly twist your torso to the right 30 to 45 degrees (or as far as you can comfortably go) so that your arms and the ball form a straight line pointing at the ground outside of your right leg.

3 In a slow, controlled manner, straighten your torso and return the ball to the center position between your legs.

4 Pause, then repeat to the left side.

Bring the ball back to center and lift the medicine ball back to start position by engaging your hamstrings and glutes to assist your lower back.

That's 1 rep.

Plank

TARGET: Gluteus maximus and minimus (glutes), erector spinae, rectus abdominis (abs), forearms, pectoralis major (pecs)

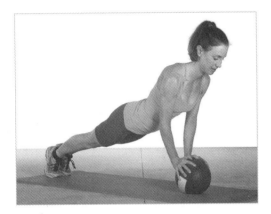

THE POSITION: From your knees, place both hands on top of a medicine ball and roll it forward to position the ball directly under your sternum (the center of your chest). Straighten your arms and legs, with the balls of your feet and toes in contact with the floor. Reposition your hands as needed to obtain a stable position. Engage your core and squeeze your glutes together to keep your spine erect and your body in a straight line from head to toe. Hold this position for as long as possible, or as required by the workout. Don't forget to breathe! If you really want to contract your abs, purse your lips and breathe as if you have a drinking straw in your mouth.

Relax and lower your knees to the floor.

Roll-Out

This is a subtle movement. The ball may move as little as an inch in either direction, though experienced athletes should shoot for more.

TARGET: Gluteus maximus and minimus (glutes), hamstrings, erector spinae, rectus abdominis (abs), forearms, pectoralis major (pecs)

STARTING POSITION: From your knees, place both hands on top of a medicine ball and roll it forward to position the ball directly under your sternum (the center of your chest). Straighten your legs, with the balls of your feet and toes in contact with the floor. Reposition your hands as needed to obtain a stable position. Engage your core and squeeze your glutes together to keep your spine erect and your body in a straight line from head to toe.

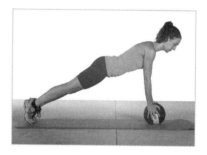

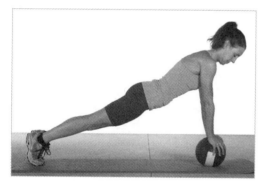

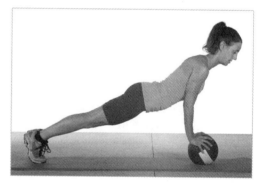

1 Using your forearms and hands, roll the ball forward (toward your head) as far as you can.

2 Bring it back to start position, then roll it backward (toward your feet) as far as you can before.

Return to start position.

One-Handed Push-Up

TARGET: Gluteus maximus and minimus (glutes), hamstrings, erector spinae, rectus abdominis (abs), obliques, forearms, triceps, biceps, pectoralis major (pecs)

STARTING POSITION: Assume a plank position (see page 66) with your right hand on the medicine ball and your left hand flat on the floor. Engage your core to keep your spine erect and keep your body in a straight line from head to toe.

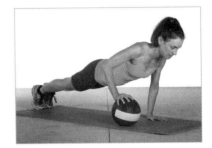

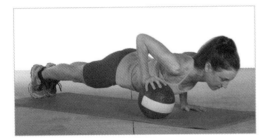

1 Inhale as you lower your upper body toward the floor, stopping when your chest touches the back of your right hand.

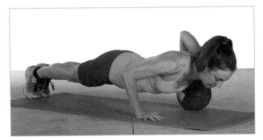

2 Using your arms, chest, back and core, exhale and push up to start position. Roll the ball to your left, switch hand positions and repeat.
That's 1 rep.

T Push-Up

TARGET: Gluteus maximus and minimus (glutes), hamstrings, erector spinae, rectus abdominis (abs), obliques, forearms, triceps, biceps, pectoralis major (pecs)

STARTING POSITION: Assume a plank position (see page 66) with your right hand on the medicine ball and your left hand flat on the floor. Engage your core to keep your spine erect and keep your body in a straight line from head to toe.

1 Inhale as you lower your upper body toward the floor, stopping when your chest touches the back of your right hand.

2 Using your arms, chest, back and core, exhale and push off the floor to return to start position, gradually transitioning your weight to your left hand while sliding your right hand under the medicine ball (you'll be cupping it in order to lift it).

3 With your left arm supporting your upper body, rotate your entire body to the right, slowly raising your right hand and pressing the ball upward until your body forms a "T." Stack your feet on top of each other if you can (stop if you experience any knee instability), maintain a contracted core and keep your spine erect. Pause.

Slowly rotate your torso back to plank position, controlling the downward motion of the medicine ball by cradling it with your right hand, then placing it on the floor. Roll the ball to your left, switch hand positions and repeat. That's 1 rep.

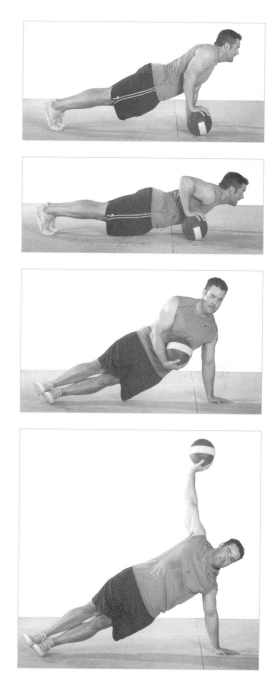

Push-Up

TARGET: Gluteus maximus and minimus (glutes), hamstrings, erector spinae, rectus abdominis (abs), obliques, forearms, triceps, biceps, pectoralis major (pecs)

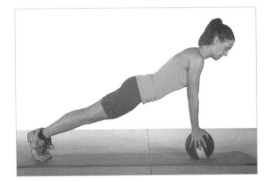

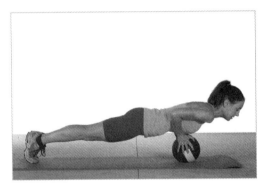

STARTING POSITION: Assume a plank position (see page 66) with both hands on either side of the medicine ball. Engage your core to keep your spine erect and keep your body in a straight line from head to toe.

1 Inhale as you lower your upper body toward the floor, stopping when your chest touches the ball.

Using your arms, chest, back and core, exhale and push up to return to start position.

Single-Arm Curl & Overhead Press

TARGET: Triceps, biceps, deltoids

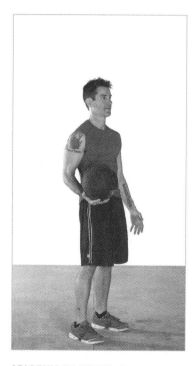
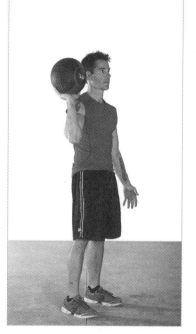
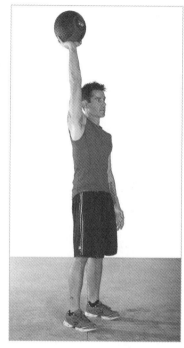

STARTING POSITION: From an athletic position, hold a medicine ball in your right hand, with your arm bent 90 degrees and your elbow and upper arm against your side, as if you were a waiter holding a plate of food in front of you.

1 Flex your biceps and raise the ball to your shoulder so your fingers are nearly touching your shoulder.

2 Press the ball directly overhead in a slow and controlled manner. Pause.

Bend your arm and carefully return the ball to your shoulder, supinate your forearm and rotate your hand with your fingers pointed away from your torso, and lower the ball slowly until your forearm is 90 degrees in relation to your upper arm.

Flip the medicine ball to your left hand (hopefully you can catch it; if not, then you may need to work on your athletic prowess a bit!), catch and repeat with your left hand. That's 1 rep.

Overhead Press & Triceps Extension

TARGET: Triceps, biceps, deltoids

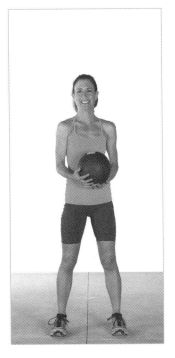 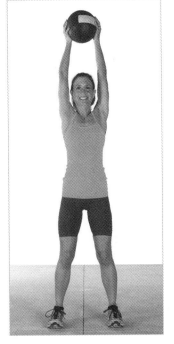 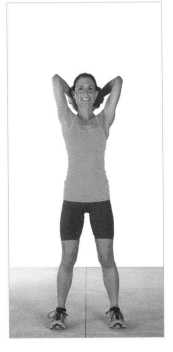

STARTING POSITION: From an athletic position, hold a medicine ball to your chest with your arms bent.

1 Press the medicine ball directly overhead until your biceps are in line with your ears. Pause.

2 Slowly lower the ball behind your head while keeping your upper arms in line with your ears. Stop before the ball touches your upper back. Pause.

Raise the ball back overhead and carefully return to start position without bonking your head, nose or chin. That's 1 rep.

Mason Twist

TARGET: Gluteus maximus and minimus (glutes), hamstrings, erector spinae, rectus abdominis (abs), obliques

STARTING POSITION: Sit on the floor with your knees comfortably bent, feet on the floor, arms bent 90 degrees and hands holding a medicine ball in front of your chest. Lift your feet about 4–6 inches off the floor and balance yourself on your posterior. Keep your core tight to protect your back.

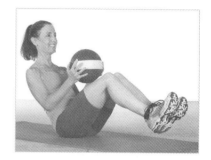

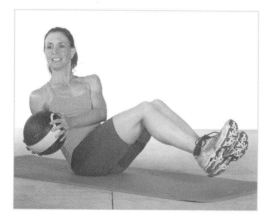

1 While maintaining the same hip position, twist your entire torso at the waist and touch the ball to the floor on the right side of your body.

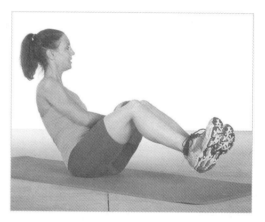

2 Keeping your feet off the floor and maintaining your balance, rotate back to center and then rotate to your left, touching the ball to the floor. Return to center. That's 1 rep.

Good Morning

TARGET: Gluteus maximus and minimus (glutes), hamstrings, erector spinae

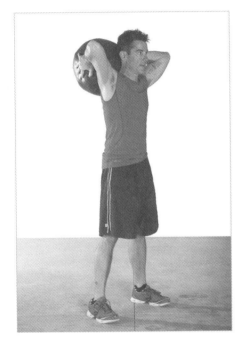

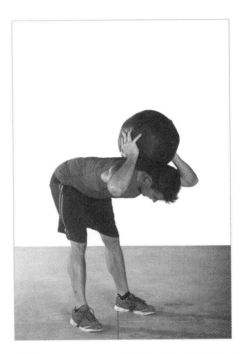

STARTING POSITION: From an athletic position, lift the medicine ball over your head and rest it carefully on the top of your back, on your spine just below your neck. Do not place the ball on your neck—the added weight on your cervical vertebrae can cause you to arch your neck, causing pain and discomfort. Steady the ball in position with your hands and bring your elbows in toward your head.

1 Keeping your core tight and back flat, bend forward at the waist until your torso is parallel to the floor. Pause.

Slowly return to start position.

Superman

Use a very light medicine ball to start.

TARGET: Gluteus maximus and minimus (glutes), erector spinae

STARTING POSITION: Lie face down on your stomach, extend your legs behind you and extend your arms directly in front of you with a medicine ball between your hands. Stretch as long as you possibly can but keep your glutes and core contracted throughout the entire movement to help stabilize your spine.

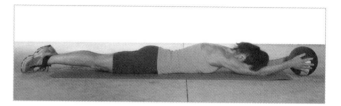

1 Gripping the medicine ball with both hands, contract your back muscles (erector spinae) and raise your arms and legs about 6–8 inches off the floor in a slow and controlled manner. Hold for 3–5 seconds.

Lower slowly back to start position.

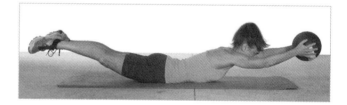

Sit-Up

If you have trouble keeping your feet on the ground, you can use a partner or a fixed object.

TARGET: Hip flexors, erector spinae, rectus abdominis (abs)

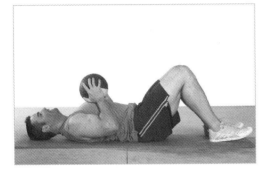

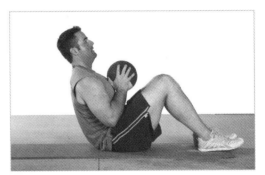

STARTING POSITION: Lie face up on the floor with your knees bent about 90 degrees. Maintain proper curvature of your lower spine, not forcing it flat to touch the floor. Hold a medicine ball in the center of your chest, with your hands on opposite sides of the ball.

1 Exhale and contract your abdominal muscles to slowly lift your head, arms and upper back off the floor in a controlled manner. Keep your upper back and neck straight and maintain your hand position on the ball through the movement. Stop when your back is at about a 45-degree angle relative to the floor. Pause briefly.

Keeping your abs tight, inhale and return to start position, lightly touching both shoulder blades to the floor. You may round your upper back slightly and roll your spine on the floor as you do so.

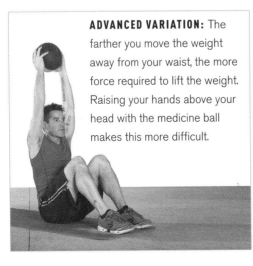

ADVANCED VARIATION: The farther you move the weight away from your waist, the more force required to lift the weight. Raising your hands above your head with the medicine ball makes this more difficult.

Ab Crunch with Toe Touch

TARGET: Hip flexors, erector spinae, rectus abdominis (abs)

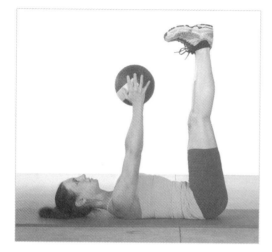

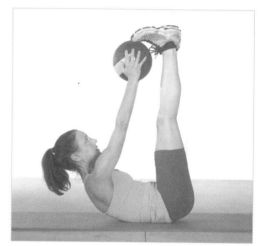

STARTING POSITION: Lie face up on the floor with your legs straight and heels pointing at the ceiling so that your body is in an "L" position. Place the medicine ball on the center of your chest, with your hands on opposite sides of it to keep it in place. Press the ball straight up toward your toes.

1 Exhale and contract your abdominal muscles to slowly lift your head, arms and upper back off the floor in a controlled manner. Keep your upper back and neck straight and maintain your hand position on the ball through the movement. Push the medicine ball upward to touch the tips of your toes. Pause briefly.

Keeping your abs tight, inhale and return to start position, lightly touching both shoulder blades to the floor. You may round your upper back slightly and roll your spine on the floor as you do so.

Figure 8

TARGET: Quadriceps femoris (quads), gluteus maximus and minimus (glutes), hamstrings, erector spinae, rectus abdominis (abs), deltoids, forearms, triceps, biceps

STARTING POSITION: From an athletic position, hold a medicine ball between both hands. Bend your waist, tilt your hips back and bend at the knees and waist as if you were performing a squat (page 54) but stop the downward motion before your upper legs are parallel with the ground. Keep your chest and head up, looking forward; don't hunch forward.

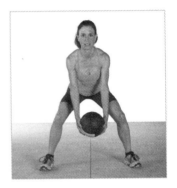

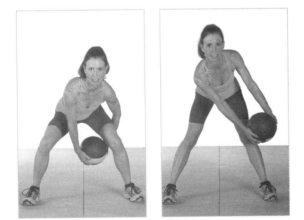

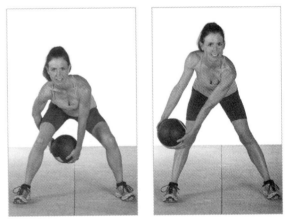

1–2 Shift the ball to your right hand and swing it around and behind your body, passing it to your left hand between your leg.

3–4 Then swing the ball around your left leg back to center, continually shifting hands and forming a figure 8.

Continue forward for the required repetitions or length of time, and then reverse directions.

Turkish Get-Up

This is a complicated move to perfect. The best way to perform this is with a training partner reading the instructions while you master the movements. Good luck!

TARGET: Full body

STARTING POSITION: Lie face up on the floor and press a medicine ball to the ceiling with your left hand. Your right arm should be extended along the floor at about 45 degrees relative to your torso. Your right leg is extended straight out from your hip, toes pointing upward. Bend your left knee and bring your left heel as close to your butt as possible, with your toe rotated outward about 5–10 degrees.

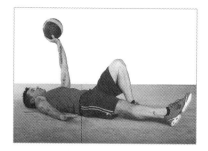

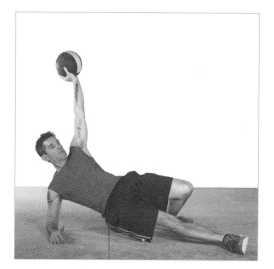

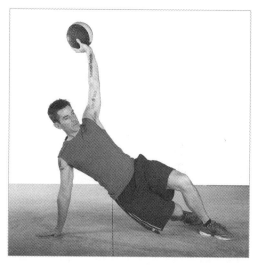

1 Press your left hand higher while rolling your torso onto your right forearm, bending at the elbow and pressing your left heel into the floor to raise your left glute off the floor while rolling onto your right hip.

2 With your left hand still holding the medicine ball, press off the floor with your right forearm and hand to straighten your right arm and place your hand on the floor; press your hips upward to lift your butt off the floor. You're now supported by your left foot flat on the ground, the outside of your right foot and your right hand.

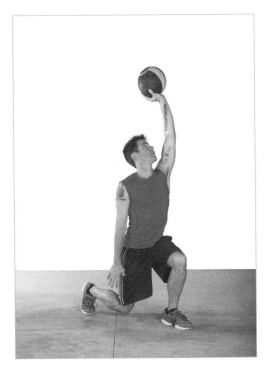

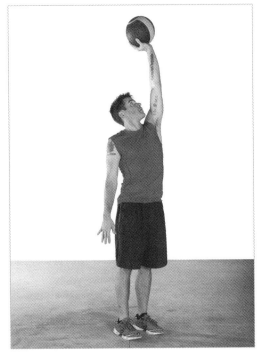

3 Bend your right knee and bring your right foot under your body, resting your weight on your right knee directly under your left hip. Push off with your right arm a little bit and rotate your torso back to square with your hips and align your knees under your hips, keeping your torso straight and perpendicular to the ground, left arm pressing the medicine ball directly overhead. Your body should look exactly like the lunge position with your left leg bent 90 degrees, foot flat on the floor, and your right leg 90 degrees with your toes and your right knee on the floor.

4 Pushing up through your left heel, straighten both knees and stand up, still keeping your left arm extended overhead with the medicine ball. Congratulations, that's exactly half of the exercise! Reverse the motion to return to start position.

Advanced Medicine Ball Exercises

These exercises are even more advanced than the Advanced program, and you won't find them in either of the workout plans in this book—that is, until you add them in! I strongly suggest that you complete both of the programs before adding these extreme medicine ball moves so you can develop the strength, flexibility, and mental acuity to perform them properly. These aren't for the faint of heart!

Pull-Up

TARGET: Trapezius, latissimus dorsi, biceps, triceps, deltoids, rectus abdominis (abs)

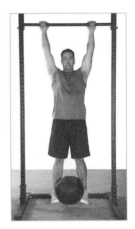

STARTING POSITION: Stand below a pull-up bar with a medicine ball on the ground between your feet. Press your feet together to pin the medicine ball between them, inhale, bend your knees and jump up and grab the bar with your preferred grip (underhand, overhand or mixed). Hang from the bar with your arms fully extended but elbows not locked.

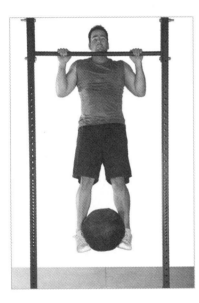

1 Squeeze your shoulder blades together (scapular retraction) to start the initial phase of the pull-up. During this initial movement, pretend that you're squeezing a pencil between your shoulder blades—don't let the pencil drop during any phase of the pull-up. Exhale and pull your chin up toward the bar by driving your elbows toward your hips. It's very important to keep your shoulders back and chest up during the entire movement. Pull yourself up in a controlled manner until the bar is just above the top of your chest.

Inhale and lower back to start position.

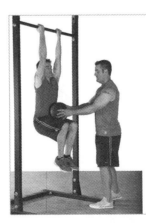

PARTNER VARIATION: Bend your knees, raise your legs 90 degrees in relation to your hips and have your partner place the medicine ball on your upper thighs.

ADVANCED VARIATION: Complete as many reps as you can without letting the ball touch the ground.

Leg Raise

TARGET: Trapezius, latissimus dorsi, biceps, triceps, rhomboids, pectoralis major (pecs), abs

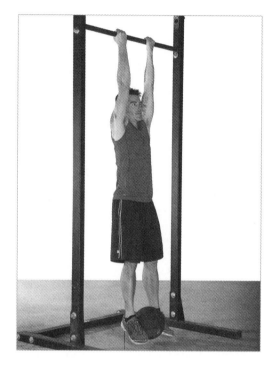 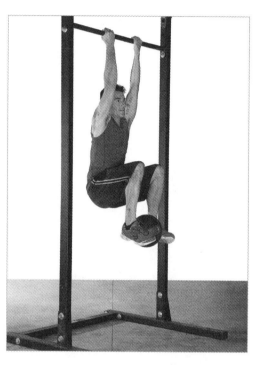

STARTING POSITION: Stand below a pull-up bar with a medicine ball on the ground between your feet. Press your feet together to pin the medicine ball between them, inhale, bend your knees and jump up and grab the bar with your preferred grip (underhand, overhand or mixed). Hang from the bar with your arms fully extended but elbows not locked.

1 Contracting your abdominal muscles, slowly bring your knees up toward your chest while keeping your torso as close to vertical as possible. Don't lean back during the movement or swing between reps. For this exercise, count 3 seconds up, hold 1–3 seconds, and then 3 seconds down.

Lower your legs in the same slow manner to start position.

Squat Jump with Foot Toss

Your feet are a bit narrower than in the goblet squat position while holding the ball, so pay extra attention to keeping your knees directly above your feet, adjusting your foot position as necessary.

TARGET: Quadriceps femoris (quads), gluteus maximus and minimus (glutes), hamstrings, erector spinae, rectus abdominis (abs), gastrocnemius (calves)

STARTING POSITION: From an athletic position, pin the medicine ball between your feet. You may need to position the ball so it's between your ankles or cradled by the tops of your feet.

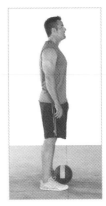

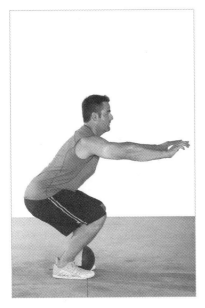

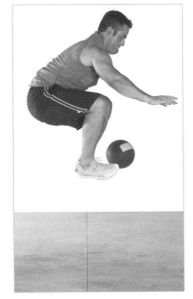

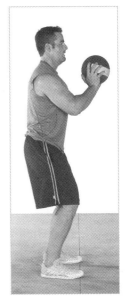

1 Inhale, bend at your hips and knees and begin to squat (see page 54). Keep your head up, eyes forward and arms out in front of you for balance. As you descend, contract your glutes while your body leans forward slightly so that your shoulders are almost in line with your knees. Continue squatting until your thighs are nearly parallel to the floor. Be careful not to let your knees roll (pronate) inward.

2–3 Swing your arms down toward the floor at your sides, driving your heels into the floor, and then explosively straighten your legs and hips and swing your arms upward in an arc directly overhead. While airborne, bend your knees and hips to rapidly "toss" the ball upward with your feet as high as possible. Lower your arms and catch the medicine ball in front of your body.

ABSOLUTELY RIDICULOUS ADVANCED VARIATION:

Not for the inexperienced—make sure you're extremely proficient at each of the advanced moves before you think about trying to pull this off. Combine these advanced moves into a "Ball Toss Pull-Up": Grab the bar with an underhand grip and perform a pull-up while tossing and catching the ball on top of (or between) your thighs. Once you figure it all out, it's a blast!

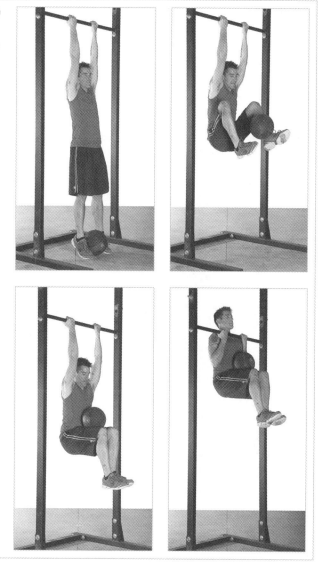

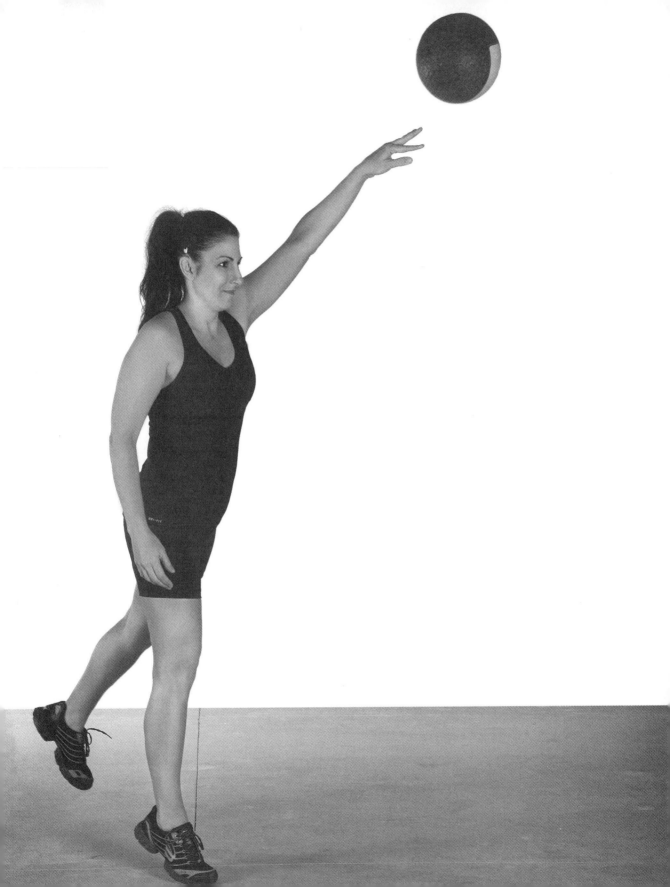

Medicine Ball Tosses

Medicine balls are a fantastic way to add weights to calisthenics but there's a lot of fun to be had just by tossing a medicine ball. Explosively throwing a medicine ball as far as you can, twisting and tossing to a partner or heaving one down against the floor or up a wall can all help to strengthen and shred your body as well as forge an iron core. And the best part? These tosses, drills and games are a blast!

Below are nine common tosses you can do with most medicine balls. Most of them will be used in various games, but each of them can be adapted to your own workout regimen by themselves. Remember, start light and stay clear of fast-moving medicine balls that are being tossed by a partner! Never try to catch a medicine ball that has been thrown a long distance—your best bet is to wait for a bounce or two before scooping it up. If you lose your balance during an overhead toss, get the heck out of the way before it comes down. A weighted sphere can do some real damage if it hits any part of your body as well as walls, ceilings and the hood of a powder blue 2007 Toyota Matrix (don't ask). Please be cautious when performing any toss or exercise!

Toss 1: Overhead Forward

With your arms extended straight overhead and the ball between both hands, keep both feet planted (no steps allowed) and pointed directly forward. Lean back slightly, engaging your core and lower back muscles. Do not bend your elbows to bring the ball behind the top of your head; your arms should always remain straight. Rapidly contract your core, bring your whole upper body forward and release the ball, bending at the waist with your follow-through. You should be throwing the ball with your core, not your arms, which should still be roughly in line with your head and neck throughout the entire motion.

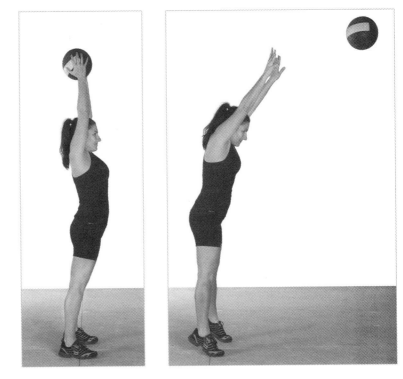

Toss 2: Underhand Forward

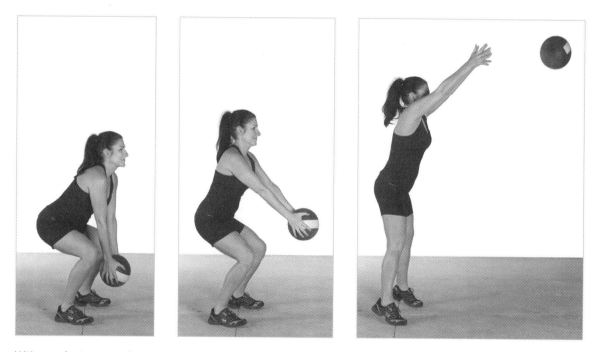

With your feet pointing forward, assume a squat position with the ball in both hands just below and in front of your knees. When you explode upward, your arms are just guiding the ball; you should be throwing the ball with the explosive force of your legs. This movement is not like a kettlebell toss—you're not swinging the ball between your legs to build momentum, but lifting and tossing from a static position. This is much harder and requires more muscle fiber recruitment to get the ball in motion and toss as far as you can.

Toss 3: Underhand Backward

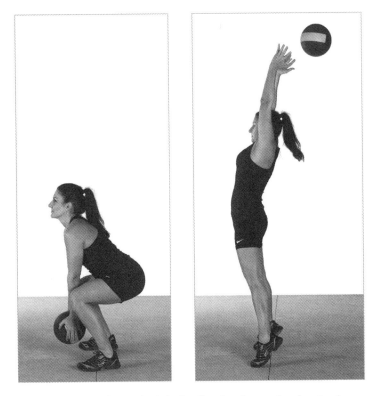

Start in a squat with your back facing the direction you're planning to throw the ball in both hands just below and in front of your knees. Explode upward, swinging your arms in an arc to lift the ball up over your head and throw it behind you. This is traditionally responsible for the longest throws and engages your entire body. Feel free to let out a strong grunt when you explode from the ground. If you're competing for distance, limit the height of the arc.

Toss 4: Shot-Put

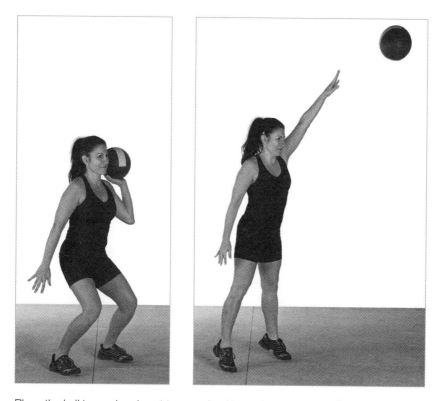

Place the ball in one hand next to your shoulder with your palm up (use your other hand to steady it if necessary). Your feet should point directly in the direction you'll be tossing. Squat straight down (don't twist) and, when you've reached the deepest part of your squat, explode upward, and toss the ball forward as far as you can. While this move uses a lot of arm muscle, you'll be using far more force from your legs to launch the ball. Alternate between hands for throws.

Toss 5: Shot-Put Twist

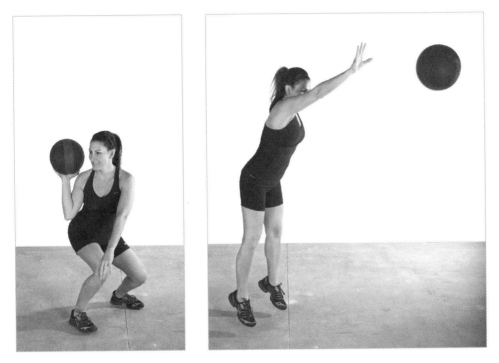

Start with your feet pointed the direction you intend to throw the ball. Hold the ball in your hand with your palm up (steady it with your other hand on the front of the ball if necessary) while you lower into a squat and twist toward the side of the hand holding the ball. At the bottom of the squat, you should have twisted far enough so that the ball is almost completely behind your body, 90 degrees in relation to the direction you'll be tossing it. Uncoil while you're exploding upward and release the ball from your hand as your chest is facing the target and your feet are pushing your entire body off the ground. This throw uses a lot of leg and arm strength, but also the torsion of your core, to chuck the ball as far as you can. Alternate between hands for throws.

Toss 6: Forward Slam

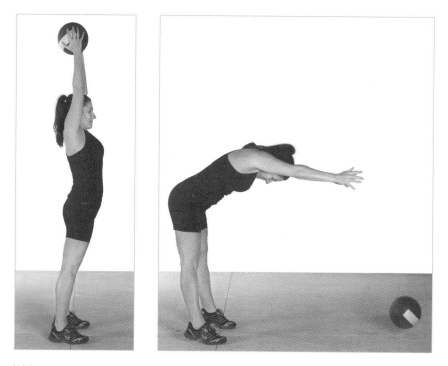

With your arms extended straight overhead with the ball between both hands, keep both feet planted (no steps allowed) and lean back slightly, engaging your core and lower back muscles. Do not bend your elbows to bring the ball behind the top of your head; your arms should always remain straight. Rapidly contract your core, bring your whole upper body forward, bending at the waist, and release the ball, throwing it as hard as you can onto the ground 6–10 feet away from your body in order to get it to bounce. You should be throwing the ball with your core, not your arms. The distance is measured by where the ball stops rolling and is traditionally one of the shorter tosses based on the bounce and roll of the ball.

Toss 7: Chest Pass

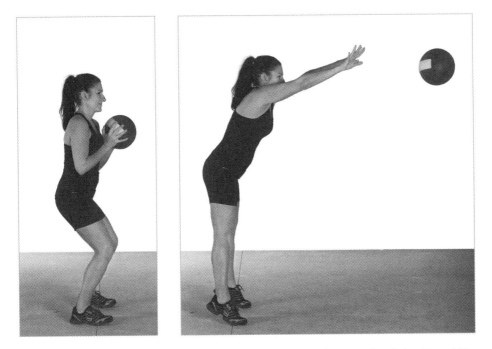

Assume an athletic stance with knees slightly bent, feet flat on the ground and shoulder-width apart, facing your target with a medicine ball at chest height. With both hands nearly on opposite sides of the ball, your right and left thumb and forefinger should be almost touching around back. Slowly bring the ball toward your upper torso until the backs of your hands touch your chest, pause and then propel the ball forward using just your arms, shoulders, chest and core to launch the ball away from you.

Toss 8: Single-Leg Shot-Put

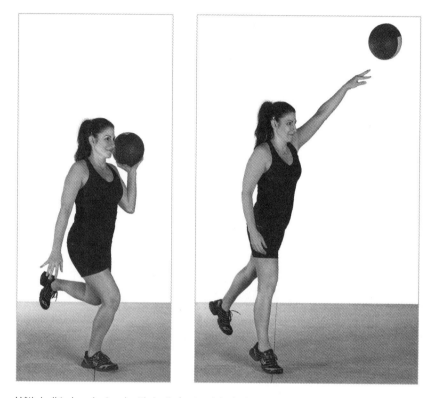

With ball in hand, stand with both feet pointed at your target and lift the foot on the same side as the hand holding the ball off the ground. Squat down as far as you can without letting your "up" foot touch the ground and launch upward from your one leg, extending your arm to release the ball. This is an excellent move to improve your balance and massively improve your core and quad strength, but also a great way to end up on your butt. This one usually takes a while to master—it's not often that you use a movement like this in daily life! Alternate between hands for each toss.

Toss 9: Hip Toss

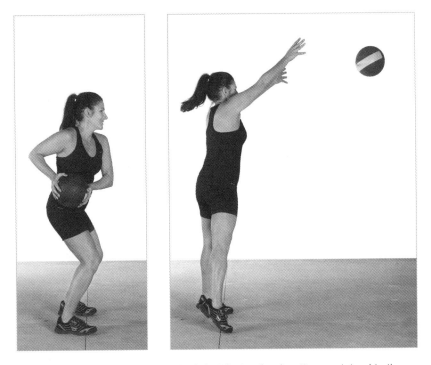

Starting in an athletic stance with both feet facing the direction you intend to throw the ball, grasp a medicine ball with both hands on opposite sides just below your waist. While keeping your hips facing your target, twist your entire torso to the right and partially extend your arms to bring the medicine ball as close to your right hip as possible. Pause, then uncoil your torso using your oblique muscles and release the ball forward as far as you can.

Games

Getting in shape is hard work; there's no real way around it. You need to eat right, exercise and recover in between workouts, not to mention try and function in your daily life. Some exercises are more enjoyable than others, but none are quite as exciting as playing competitive games with yourself or a partner. Whether you're on your own or facing off against a friendly opponent, challenge yourself with these games by giving your all to each sprint, lift, carry or toss and you'll reap the endurance, strength, speed and weight-loss benefits. These games were designed to enhance athletic performance and erase the doldrums and monotony of plain old cardio while using medicine ball tosses, lifts and carries. They'll augment squats and sprints to stoke your metabolism, torch fat and build a lean, strong physique. "Toss and Run" was actually inspired by and adapted from an exercise performed at some NFL training camps to build functional strength, develop a strong core and support muscles for the rigors of a football season.

Toss & Run

Number of players: 1

DESCRIPTION: Throw a medicine ball as far as possible using an underhand technique. Once the ball is released, sprint after it as fast as you can. Gather the medicine ball and throw again until you've reached the end of the field. Repeat with no rest, going back down the field to the starting position. Alternate through tosses 1, 2, 4, 6, 7 and 9. Repeat until you're exhausted. Enjoy!

Leapfrog

There's no real winner or loser in this game as far as points go—both you and your partner will have to be content with just getting a great sprint-and-toss workout.

Number of players: 2

DESCRIPTION: Both players start at an end line on a football or soccer field or a cone placed on a flat stretch of grass at least 50 yards long (the longer the better!). One person starts the game by throwing the medicine ball as far as possible using an overhand forward toss. Both players sprint after the ball as soon as it's released. The non-tossing player gathers the ball and throws it farther down the field. The original tosser will already be sprinting past him to catch up with the ball as it lands, setting their feet and launching back into the air before breaking back into a sprint. During this fast-paced game, alternate through tosses 1, 2, 4, 6, 7 and 9 each time you pick up the ball. Also, make sure you alternate sides with the shot-put toss and hip toss. Always make sure you're throwing the ball straight ahead and not at your partner's back! You should be spaced wide enough that the medicine ball will not strike either of you while you're running.

Out & Back Sprints

When's the last time you sprinted with a medicine ball overhead? Well, in this game, your goal is to exhaust the other player by throwing the ball as far as you can with each toss. You'd better make sure they're tired out because they'll be doing the same to you!

Number of players: 1, 2 (2-person description below, can be modified for solo game)

DESCRIPTION: Start with 2 players side by side at a pair of cones. One player tosses the ball, alternating between an overhand forward, underhand forward, shot-put, chest or hip toss. For the shot-put and hip tosses, make sure to switch sides between rounds. Once the ball is released, the other player sprints after the ball, picks it up over his head and sprints back with the ball overhead. Be careful and keep a good grip on the ball over your head. When the sprinter makes it back to the starting position, switch roles (if you have more than 2 players, just rotate so everyone gets a turn). Win the game by being the last one standing!

Distance Tosses

The goal is to create as much distance between your partner's cones by tossing a medicine ball back and forth using a variety of throwing techniques. This involves a lot of jumping, squatting and twisting, so make sure you're warmed up before attempting any of them.

SAFETY NOTE: *NEVER try to catch a thrown medicine ball that has been thrown with high velocity. Stand out of the way and let it bounce!*

Number of players: 1, 2 (2-person description below, can be modified for solo game)

DESCRIPTION: Using 4 cones, place 2 cones side by side and the other pair about 10 feet away. Stand next to a pair of cones and face your partner, who's standing next to the other pair of cones. Choose who goes first. Begin tossing the ball as far as you can toward your partner's cones. Your partner will move his "distance cone" (just pick one of the cones to move) to the spot where your ball bounces. In the case of the forward slam, it'll be where the ball finishes rolling. Your opponent will make his next throw from there, whether it's farther or closer than the original 10 feet. The "starting cone" will remain in place to mark the spot from which you began the match. A match is played by alternating through all 9 tosses starting on page 87 to determine a winner for each round. The winner is the person whose distance cone is still closest to his starting cone.

Cross-Ball

This game started out pretty simply as two players trying to toss a light (4- or 6-pound) medicine ball past each other within the confines of a "goal" made up by 2 cones. Immediately, it was a hit and Jason (author of Ultimate Jump Rope Workouts*) and I started playing a ton of matches daily and refined the rules in a whole host of ways. We developed penalties, different scoring plays and even a round-robin tournament with multiple players on each team where the action never stopped. Maybe in retrospect we loved the game a little too much and tinkered with the rules a little too often. So here it is in the original form. If you'd like to expand on it, then have a blast.*

ALLOWED TOSSES: Shot-Put, Chest Pass, Hip Toss, Underhand Forward

PLEASE NOTE: There's some risk associated with this game since you and a partner will be heaving a medicine ball toward each other with the intention of catching it off the bounce. Overhand forward and underhand backward are too dangerous to be used in this type of game as the ball can be thrown with high velocity. Only use the allowed tosses and be cautious—this game is for fun and fitness, not trying to hurt each other! Always be careful when catching a bounced medicine ball as you can easily injure your hands, arms or any part of your body that unintentionally comes in contact with the ball. Never try to catch a ball that has not bounced in the field of play.

DESCRIPTION: Set up 2 goals with cones 12 feet apart from each other—this area is the field of play. Both goals should be 8 feet wide. The goal is to toss the ball so that it bounces in the field of play and then through the opponent's goal; the opponent's goal is to catch the ball with both hands before it touches the ground inside their goal. There is no point scored unless the ball touches the ground, despite bouncing over the goal line.

All tosses take place from each goal line; there's no stepping forward into the field of play in order to toss the ball. That's a foul and the ball is turned over to the opponent.

SCORING:

- 1 point if ball bounces in the field of play and then touches the ground on the opposite side of the opponent's goal line

- 1 point for opponent if you toss the ball over their goal line without it bouncing in the field of play

- 1 point for opponent if you toss or bounce the ball out of bounds on the outside of either of your opponent's goal cones. The first one to 5 points wins.

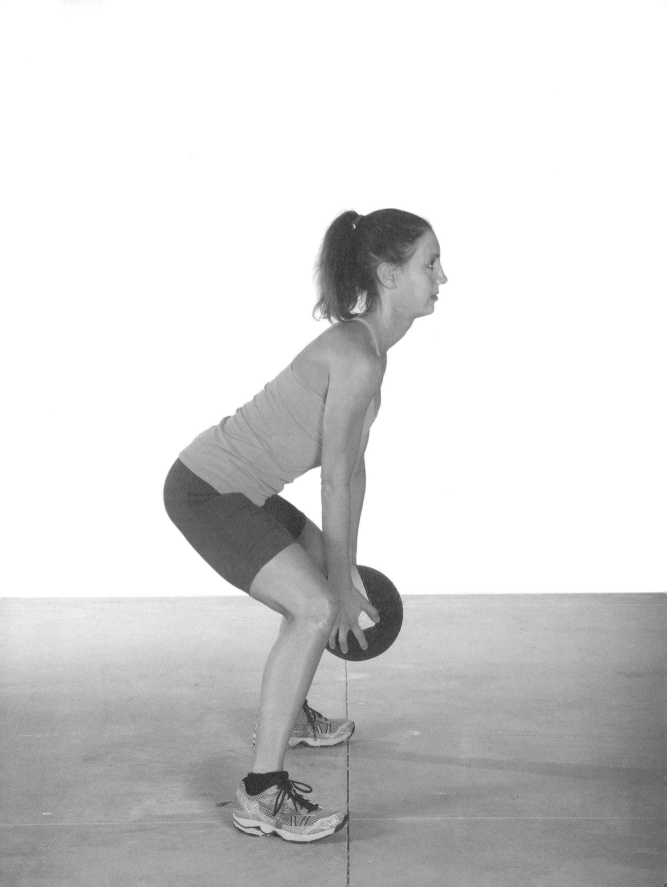

PART 4: APPENDIX

Warming Up & Stretching

Prior to your workout, you'll want to warm up and loosen any tight muscles—but not put them through any rigorous stretching as that can wreak havoc on cold, inflexible muscle fibers. Stretches are to be performed only on warm muscles, optimally after you've completed your workout, in order to promote blood flow and speed up healing (and growing). A good stretch is one where you extend the muscle and work it through a full range of motion, and the stretch should be a slow and controlled movement—never bounce!

Once you've completed a basic warm-up (like 5 minutes of walking on a treadmill or elliptical, 50 jumping jacks, 50 toe touches or similar), use the "Dynamic Yoga Warm-Up" on page 104. This sequence of movements will get your lower body ready.

POOR MAN'S YOGA DYNAMIC WARM-UP

"Dynamic Yoga Warm-Up" on page 104 is called the "Poor Man's Yoga" sequence because it's a combination of moves that requires balance, flexibility and strength while providing great post–warm-up dynamic activation of your lower body and core. This sequence will get the muscles and joints of your lower body ready for the workout and will make sure your muscles, tendons and ligaments have full range of motion and sufficient pliability for your workout. Remember, this isn't a stretch per se; it's a fluid series of sequential movements to work your body on multiple planes using multiple muscles across multiple joints—the true definition of a dynamic compound movement. Be sure to perform each movement carefully and correctly to maximize the benefits. I greatly recommend that you practice all three of these moves by themselves before you do them in combination, especially the lunge. Like any other exercise, performing warm-ups, stretches or dynamic movements like these is a complete waste of time and can potentially cause an injury if done with bad form. Bad lunge form can cause you to bow your upward knee inward and potentially damage your knee—bad news. Plus, you may need to build up your balance from position to position in order to maintain proper form. Take your time, learn how to do it right and then worry about adding intensity or frequency. Don't rush movements simply to move on; just

> **TIP:** Walk to the gym if you can. One to two miles of walking will raise your body temperature, engage your core and warm up your legs. Aside from the physical benefits, this is a great way to clear your mind and mentally prepare before a workout and to cool down and loosen up tight muscles on your way home.

focus on doing them correctly and it will become second nature.

After you've completed the "yoga" sequence, be sure to also warm up your upper body. Work through the movements on pages 106 to 108 to prepare your arms, shoulders, chest and back. These exercises also serve as great stretches for your entire body after you're done with your workout.

Dynamic Yoga Warm-Up

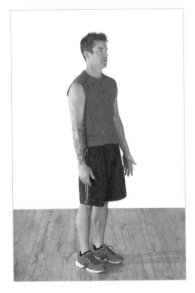 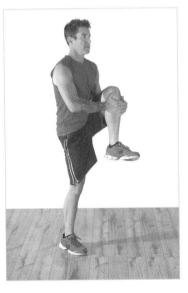 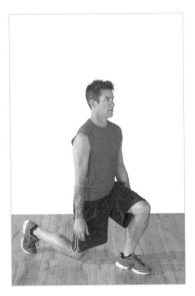

1 Stand up straight in an athletic stance, with shoulders back, head high, back straight, hands at sides, knees slightly bent and feet about shoulder-width apart with toes pointed slightly outward.

2 Shift your weight to your right foot while bending your left knee and bringing it up toward your chest. Place your hands on your upper shin, below your knee, and slowly apply force to bring your knee closer to your upper torso while maintaining your balance. Release your left leg if you lose your balance; do not allow your right knee to bow inward or outward as it may result in injury.

3 Keeping your upper body upright, your head high, shoulders back and core braced to keep your back straight, slowly, in a controlled manner, release your hands and step forward about 2 feet with your left foot and place it on the ground. Drop your hips straight down into a lunge position. Your left leg should be bent 90 degrees, with your upper leg parallel with the ground and lower leg perpendicular to it; your right toes should be on the ground with your right leg also bent 90 degrees.

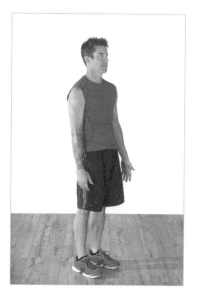

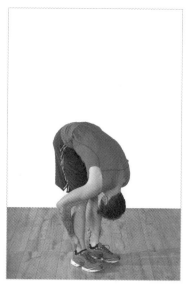

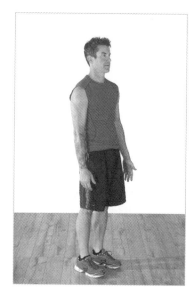

4 Slowly press up from your left heel and push your body back into a standing position with both feet parallel.

5 Bend at the waist and bring your head toward your knees, placing your hands on the backs of your lower calves and pulling slightly to assist in getting your noggin closer to your knees.

6 Release your hands and slowly return to starting position. That's 1 rep.

Repeat with your right leg. Perform 5 reps on each side. Never bounce or yank with your arms to pull yourself into position. As you repeat, each subsequent movement should provide a little deeper range of motion.

Arms across Chest

THE STRETCH: Stand with your feet shoulder-width apart. Bring your left arm across your chest. Support your left elbow with the crook of your right arm by raising your right arm and bending it 90 degrees. Gently pull your left arm to your chest while maintaining proper posture (straight back, wide shoulders). Don't round or hunch your shoulders. Hold your arm to your chest for 10 seconds.

Release and switch arms. After you've done both sides, shake your hands out for 5–10 seconds.

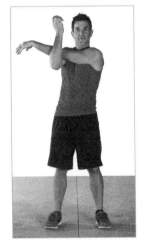

Chest

THE STRETCH: Clasp your hands together behind your lower back with palms facing each other. Keeping an erect posture and your arms as straight as possible, gently pull your arms away from your back straight out behind you. Keep your shoulders down. Hold for 10 seconds.

Rest for 30 seconds and repeat.

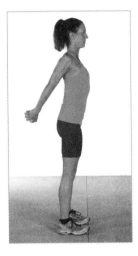

Shoulders & Upper Back

THE STRETCH: Stand with your feet shoulder-width apart and extend both arms straight out in front of you. Interlace your fingers and turn your palms to face away from your body. Keeping your back straight, exhale and reach your palms away from your body, pushing through your shoulders and upper back. Allow your neck to bend naturally as you round your upper back. Continue to reach your hands and stretch for 10 seconds.

Rest for 30 seconds then repeat. After you've done the second set, shake your arms out to your sides for 10 seconds to return blood to the fingers and forearm muscles.

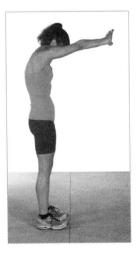

Arm Circles

1-3 Stand with your feet shoulder-width apart. Move both arms in a complete circle forward 5 times and then backward 5 times.

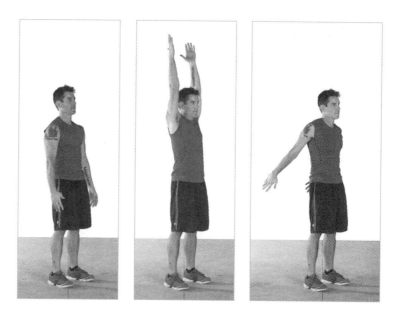

Around the World

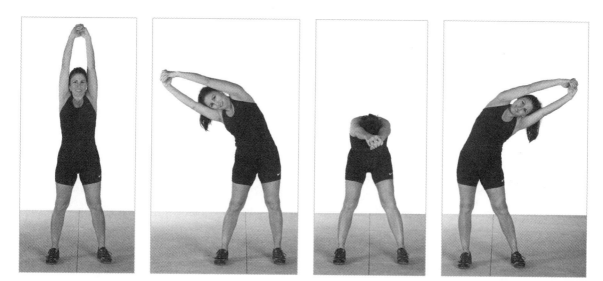

1 Stand with your feet shoulder-width apart and extend your hands overhead with elbows locked, fingers interlocked and palms up. Keep your arms straight the entire time.

2-4 Bending at the hips, bring your hands down toward your right leg and, in a continuous circular motion, bring your hands toward your toes, then toward your left leg and then return your hands overhead and bend backward.

Repeat 3 times then change directions.

Lumberjack

1 Stand with your feet shoulder-width apart and extend your hands overhead with elbows locked, fingers interlocked and palms up.

2 Bend forward at the waist and try to put your hands on the ground (like you're chopping wood).

Raise up and repeat.

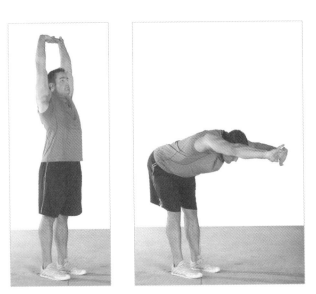

Child's Pose

THE POSITION: From a kneeling position, sit your butt back on your calves, then lean forward and place your lower torso on your thighs. Extend your arms directly out in front of you, parallel to each other, and lower your chest toward the floor. Reach your arms as far forward as you can, and rest your forearms and hands flat on the floor. Hold for 30 seconds.

Release and then rest for 10 seconds.

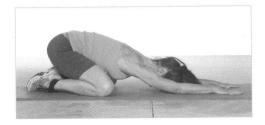

Cobra

This stretches and strengthens your abs and back and is a great way to cool down between sets of multiple repetitions.

THE POSITION: Lying on your stomach, place your hands directly under your shoulders with your fingers facing forward. Straighten your legs and point your toes. Exhale and engage your core while lifting your chest off the floor and pushing your hips gently into the floor. Your arms help guide you through the movement, and your elbows should remain slightly bent at the top of the extension; your hips should remain in contact with the mat. Hold the "up" position for 15–30 seconds, then gently roll your upper body back to the floor.

Rest for 10 seconds.

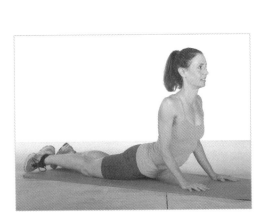

Index

Acknowledgments

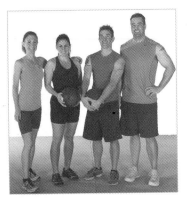

Tricia Schafer, Kristen Stewart, Brett Stewart and Jason Warner

A huge thanks to our models (Tricia Schafer, Jason Warner and Kristen Stewart) and photographer Scott Whitney for putting up with my crazy schedule and showing up nearly anytime, anywhere to get the shot!

Special thanks to Claire and Chris Treanor from CrossFit Blade in Phoenix, Arizona, Brian Peitz of Fuzion Fitness in Phoenix and Glendale, Arizona, Jimbeau Andrews from Ryders Eyewear, and Andy Krafsur from Spira Footwear for their continued support.

Special thanks and belated apologies to Michael Bennett, my marathon, ultramarathon and Ironman training partner, teammate, photographer and friend. I'm really sorry you misjudged the bounce of that medicine ball back in 2010 and broke your rib a few weeks before P.F. Chang's Rock 'N' Roll Marathon. Now, can you never bring that up again as an excuse for your slowest marathon time ever?

Of course, how could I ever write this book without everything I learned from Jason Warner, my co-author for *Ultimate Jump Rope Workouts*, *7 Weeks to 10 Pounds of Muscle*, and contributor to nearly all my other books including *7 Weeks to Getting Ripped*, where a lot of the ideas and exercises in this book got their start.

All my love and heartfelt thanks to my family and friends for their support. (My parents and brother are pretty awesome.) Vivi and Ian, I love you both very much and am so proud to be your dad. Kristen, I still can't figure out why you love me so much, but far be it for me to question the best thing that has ever happened to a geek like me.

About the Author

Brett Stewart is a certified personal trainer, a running and triathlon coach, and an endurance athlete who currently resides in Phoenix, Arizona. An avid multisport athlete, Brett has completed dozens of triathlons, marathons, ultramarathons and obstacle races. He's constantly looking for new fitness challenges and developing new workouts and routines for himself, his friends and his clients. Brett can be contacted at www.7weekstofitness.com and is available for speaking at corporate wellness and fitness events across the United States.